A Guide to Supporting Breastfeeding for the Medical Profession

This book is a practical guide for medical practitioners as they navigate through breastfeeding problems that occur in day-to-day practice.

If mothers have a breastfeeding complication they are often directed to their GP. In complex situations, medical staff will be making decisions around what treatment plan to follow and whether a mother can keep breastfeeding. In recent years there has been growing evidence that medical professionals often advise mothers to stop breastfeeding while undergoing treatment, when in reality this was not a necessary step. In a time when breastfeeding rates are decreasing, it is important that medical professionals give accurate advice and support a mother's choice to breastfeed if the situation allows it. *A Guide to Supporting Breastfeeding for the Medical Profession* includes contributions from a wide range of medical professionals and each chapter is written with the practitioner in mind. Contributors include GPs, paediatricians, neonatologists, lactation specialists and midwives.

Doctors have a vital role to play in supporting and facilitating breastfeeding, and without the appropriate knowledge they can often inadvertently sabotage it. This book will be of interest to GPs and paediatricians as well as nurse prescribers, midwives and health visitors.

Amy Brown is Professor of Child Public Health at Swansea University, where she has published over 100 research papers and books examining psychological, cultural and societal barriers to breastfeeding. Her research seeks to shift our perception of breastfeeding from an individual mothering issue to a wider public health challenge.

Wendy Jones is a pharmacist, with over 25 years of experience as a breastfeeding support worker for the Breastfeeding Network (BfN). She runs the BfN Drugs in Breastmilk Service and has presented widely to healthcare professionals, volunteers and mothers on this subject. She qualified as an independent pharmacist prescriber but is now retired.

A Guide to Supporting Breastfeeding for the Medical Profession

Edited by Amy Brown and Wendy Jones

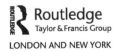

LONDON AND NEW YORK

First published 2020
by Routledge
2 Park Square, Milton Park, Abingdon, Oxon OX14 4RN

and by Routledge
52 Vanderbilt Avenue, New York, NY 10017

Routledge is an imprint of the Taylor & Francis Group, an informa business

British Library Cataloguing-in-Publication Data
A catalogue record for this book is available from the British Library

Library of Congress Cataloging-in-Publication Data
A catalog record has been requested for this book

ISBN: 978-0-367-20644-4 (hbk)
ISBN: 978-0-367-20646-8 (pbk)
ISBN: 978-0-429-26269-2 (ebk)

Typeset in Sabon
by Newgen Publishing UK

Contents

vi *Contents*

Figures

Tables

Foreword

There is extensive and resounding evidence that breastfeeding saves lives, improves health and cuts costs in every country worldwide, rich and poor alike.

However, breastfeeding is an emotive issue in the UK, because so many families have not breastfed, or have experienced the trauma of trying very hard to breastfeed and not succeeding. We need to shift the conversation around breastfeeding away from guilt and blame; it is not individual mothers' responsibility to tackle an entrenched public health issue. To ensure best outcomes for babies, their mothers and families, we must work to remove the myriad of barriers to breastfeeding in the UK – social, cultural, economic, physical and practical – to help mothers to breastfeed for as long as they wish.

A key part of this work involves improving healthcare support around infant feeding. We know that families need consistent, face-to-face, evidence-based guidance about feeding, and the Baby Friendly Initiative's work has helped support this provision in maternity and community services. However, looking beyond maternity units and community services, one of the most common complaints we hear from mothers is that they have received inconsistent information from other health professionals caring for them. This feedback demonstrates how important it is for us to take a wider view of breastfeeding support. Historically, health professionals who weren't routinely involved in the care of newborns received very little formal education on why breastfeeding is important and how to support families with feeding – now this is changing, and the need for all professionals to understand breastfeeding is becoming increasingly recognised. We still have a long way to go before the health service as a whole, from GPs to dieticians, is empowered to support breastfeeding, but books like this demonstrate that we are moving in the right direction.

We urge the UK and devolved governments to take action to create a supportive, enabling environment for women who want to breastfeed. This should involve developing a National Infant Feeding Strategy to show leadership in breastfeeding protection; supporting breastfeeding in all relevant policy areas, from obesity to school readiness; implementing evidence-based initiatives that support breastfeeding; and protecting the public from harmful commercial interests by adopting, in full, the International Code of Marketing of Breastmilk Substitutes and subsequent resolutions. Only by taking such a holistic approach can we implement long-lasting change for women who want to breastfeed.

We welcome this book in its recognition of the need to better support our health professionals, so that they are all enabled to provide high-quality infant feeding care.

Sue Ashmore, Programme Director, Unicef UK Baby Friendly Initiative

Acknowledgements

The development of this book stemmed from a comment made to Amy by a breastfeeding expert during the evaluation of the Breastfeeding Network Drugs in Breastmilk Helpline. 'We really need a book to help professionals understand more about breastfeeding', she said. This sparked the first thoughts about how this could be achieved and what we hope to accomplish by producing it.

Our thoughts immediately turned to our friends, the experts in so many aspects of breastfeeding specialities. They could write the information on their specialist topics so much better than we could. Most generously, they all agreed. Routledge were receptive to the idea and so began the crazy last few months that we have spent talking about breastfeeding even more than usual. We wrote our own chapters and edited the ones so kindly written by our associates. We learned even more along the way about how special breastmilk is and how strong breastfeeding mothers can be.

Along the way the Unicef Baby Friendly Initiative began work on the suite of learning outcomes to support new healthcare practitioners involved in the care for new babies, their mothers and families in UK public services. We believe that this book underpins these and will become the basis for future professionals and an opportunity for continued professional development in those of us already qualified and working with families.

We would like to dedicate this book to our own families who always support us with patience as we write, and to the many thousands of mothers and professionals who contact both of us each year to ask about breastfeeding. We cannot begin to express our gratitude to the contributors to this book; thank you doesn't seem enoughm but we think you know how much we value your knowledge.

The final benefactor of this book will be the Human Milk Foundation (www. hunanmilkfoundation.org) whose aim is to provide milk for all babies as well as to continue research. All royalties from the sales of this book will go directly to them, helping them to continue their work.

1 The role of primary care and the GP in supporting breastfeeding

Marie-Therese Lovis

The fact that you are reading this book suggests you are probably already convinced that the primary care team has a role in supporting breastfeeding. This chapter overviews

- the benefits of breastfeeding for mothers, babies and you;
- reassuring mothers about what is normal;
- strategies that you can put in place to help support breastfeeding;
- counselling mothers who want to stop breastfeeding.

Sometimes it is a lonely place convincing others that the primary care team should support breastfeeding. It is widely acknowledged that there is a significant learning need around infant feeding within primary and secondary care (Renfrew et al. 2006). In this chapter I will therefore focus on giving you some tools to change the environment of the surgery, surgery communications, engagement of clinicians and resources available. If you need a hook to get the attention of the most reluctant of colleagues, perhaps share with them that the Care Quality Commission looks favourably on practices that are breastfeeding-friendly. You could also share the data that show that if we were able to increase breastfeeding rates to enable those exclusively breastfeeding at 1 week to continue to 4 months, we could save 11 million NHS pounds. This saving includes a significant reduction in GP appointments through a reduction in common childhood respiratory and gastrointestinal infections (Pokhrel et al. 2015). I don't know about your surgery, but I could do with an extra 15% of appointments to offer my patients!

I will approach the role of primary care by following the patient journey and all that could be done for that patient to support breastfeeding. Please note this is not about forcing mothers to breastfeed when they do not wish to but is about supporting every mother to breastfeed her child for as long as she wishes to.

When mothers, particularly first-time mothers, venture out after the birth of a baby, the concern about breastfeeding in public can be a real issue for some. A practice can do much to support mothers to breastfeed outside the home. A simple gesture of posters in the waiting room or on your waiting-room screens advising 'you are welcome to breastfeed here' can go a long way. Posters can be easily printed off from the Unicef Baby Friendly Initiative website.

Breastfeeding mothers are protected by the UK Equality Act 2010 which defines treating a woman unfavourably because she is breastfeeding as discrimination. A mother breastfeeding at a GP surgery is therefore protected by Equality Law (unless there are health and safety risks, e.g. you might legitimately ask a breastfeeding mother to move to an isolation room if she or her infant has chickenpox or measles). It is useful to share this legislation with your reception staff as they will be the mother's first-line defence against members of the public who may wish to make abusive comments to the mother about feeding elsewhere or about her to staff or others. A simple statement from reception that the mother is entitled by law to feed her baby in the waiting room will support a mother. It is also important to educate all patient-facing staff about infant feeding as simple gestures such as offering a glass of water to a breastfeeding mother on a hot day can make her feel supported by your team. Educating the whole team can also help to stop staff giving anecdotal advice to mothers that is at odds with NHS guidance and evidence.

Some mothers do wish to breastfeed somewhere more private, particularly if they are having struggles to establish a good latch or just if the baby has got to an age where s/he is more interested in the surroundings than feeding. If space permits, it is useful to be able to offer a simple private area for mothers to breastfeed if they prefer, perhaps with a box of tissues and wipe-clean toys in a box for an accompanying toddler. Think about where this might be and about visibility from windows and accessibility with a buggy. If you do not have space for a designated breastfeeding area, it can be useful for reception to have an awareness of any rooms that may be unoccupied (and with desks clear of clinical and patient-identifying information) so that a mother can be shown to a room to feed. Think about the language you use to advertise this space to ensure that it does not imply that mothers must feed in a designated area.

When you call a mother into the clinical room, if you see that she is feeding you could offer to let her finish the feed and see your next patient first if she wishes. The language that we use can have wide-reaching impacts on a mother's breastfeeding journey. The simple question, 'Are you *still* breastfeeding?' has a value statement embedded in it, and whether you internally are thinking, 'That is great that she is still feeding' or 'Why is she bothering to breastfeed still?' the patient may well hear the latter value judgement. I would urge you to be curious but simple in your questions. 'Are you breastfeeding?' will suffice. Nine out of ten women in one study reported that they stopped breastfeeding before they wanted to (Bolling et al. 2007). Some of the factors listed in their reasons for this were that they were advised to stop by a professional. As primary care clinicians we can have a profound impact on that mother's breastfeeding journey.

Within the consultation there are so many instances when we can support rather than undermine the breastfeeding dyad as a GP/primary care clinician and these might include signposting to a feeding assessment for all mothers presenting with mastitis. Antibiotics are not first-line in the first 24 hours in an otherwise well mother, and improving latch may help prevent further episodes. At every contact, praise the mother for every drop of breast milk she gives to her baby, via whatever means. In our formula-feeding culture there are few cheerleaders out there for the breastfeeding mother. As a health professional your words carry significant weight in helping that mother feel that what she is doing is worthwhile.

Discussions with patients about a perceived need to stop breastfeeding

When mothers say to me, 'I have to stop breastfeeding because I'm going back to work,' I would first check, 'Do you want to stop breastfeeding or would you prefer to continue if you could?' If they say that they want to continue I share that I have returned to work from 7 months with my four children and have pumped at work. I have fed my children for a range of 7 months to 3 years for varying reasons according to what felt right for us at the time. 'Would you like to know more about expressing breastmilk or tips for returning to work and continuing to breastfeed?' then allows further discussion about the practicalities, which if you are not able to give you could then signpost to a resource such as a breastfeeding support phone line (e.g. National Breastfeeding Helpline: 03001000212, 9.30 a.m. to 9.30 p.m., which also has a web chat service).

It can also be useful to signpost to employment support in regard to their rights on return to work: https://maternityaction.org.uk/advice/continuing-to-breastfeed-when-you-return-to-work/. Whilst we are on this subject, are you aware that the NHS has clear guidelines on supporting employees returning to work breastfeeding? Do you have a practice policy on supporting your colleagues when they return to work? Do you discuss where and when they will have opportunities to express milk and offer safe storage of expressed milk until the end of their working day?

Some women think they need to stop breastfeeding either permanently or due to advice to 'pump and dump' due to medication that they are on. Ensure you are up to date in your advice. The LactMed app is useful to have on your phone for quick evidence around safety in breastfeeding. Online resources include the UK Drugs in Lactation Advisory Service (UKDILAS; www.sps.nhs.uk/articles/ukdilas/), an NHS prescribing advisory service and the Breastfeeding Network website (www.breastfeedingnetwork. org.uk/detailed-information/drugs-in-breastmilk/), which has great patient information leaflets on a range of medications and their use in breastfeeding mothers. I find it useful to pre-empt queries from well-meaning community pharmacists by printing e.g. the metronidazole leaflet and giving it to the patient as I have found that, unhelpfully, the *British National Formulary* (BNF) flags it as unsuitable in breastfeeding and so pharmacists have on occasion refused to dispense. Furthermore, cite the leaflet in the medical notes so that colleagues who see the patient after you, and who may not be as versed as you in prescribing in breastfeeding, can be empowered to support rather than undermine your advice.

Recognising and reassuring regarding normality

Be clear about what is within the physiological norm and be empowered to reassure when that is so. Online forums may advise mum that baby clearly has reflux or cows' milk allergy and that can make it difficult to have that conversation when the parents' expectations are set at the start of the consultation. There is no denying the effects on parents of the sleepless nights, extra washing and general relentlessness that having a tiny human who vomits or cries a lot can bring. It is so important to check in with the mental health of both parents. Mental health issues can underlie a concern about infant feeding, reflux or crying; living with a baby who cries a lot can also impact on mental health. You may find the Royal College of General Practitioners' perinatal mental health toolkit a useful resource for supporting both parents – www.rcgp. org.uk/clinical-and-research/resources/toolkits/perinatal-mental-health-toolkit.aspx. http://purplecrying.info/ is a useful website to reassure about the utterly normal, yet absolutely difficult, phase commonly known as 'colic'. Sometimes just knowing that 'this too shall pass' can be helpful, as well as managing expectations regarding what they thought parenthood and breastfeeding might look like and the realities. This can include managing expectations of breastfeeding and the frequency with which infants do need to feed. In today's society of instant responses and increased control over our lives, tiny humans can provoke confusion in their grown-ups as they regularly demonstrate that they have not read the memo regarding Western cultural expectations of them and remind us of their biologically driven need for warmth, physical contact, regular nutrition and regular sleep with regular wakenings that protect them from sudden infant death syndrome and a need via all of the above for assistance with regulation of homeostasis whilst their bodies develop.

Continuing the theme of normality, it is useful to be able to give evidence-based advice and support around sleep issues. www.basisonline.org.uk/ is a great resource for parents and professionals that can help arm parents against the onslaught of friendly advice that if they only give a bottle baby will sleep through the night (this myth is not supported by the evidence). Of note, in terms of 'sleeping through the night', in medical terms this is classed as 5 hours: this might help manage expectations.

First do no harm. It is of course important to diagnose cows' milk protein allergy or gastro-oestophageal reflux disease where it is present and provide evidence-based treatment and support for the family. There are also real dangers to overdiagnosing medical conditions and to overprescribing. These dangers include risking the breastfeeding journey and all the subsequent risks of not breastfeeding, as outlined in the *Lancet* breastfeeding series 2016 (www.thelancet.com/series/breastfeeding), risks to baby from unnecessary exclusion diets or medication and risks to the mother, including risks to her mental health if she stops breastfeeding sooner than she had intended. Recent studies have shown concerns around a significant increase in fracture risk in children who received proton pump inhibitors and H2 antagonists in the first 6 months of life. Gaviscon is commonly found to cause constipation in infants and mothers report that it can be difficult to give to a breastfed baby.

If you do diagnose delayed cows' milk protein allergy then it is important to encourage continued breastfeeding as per the 2019 iMAP guidelines, now hosted by the GP Infant Feeding Network website (https://gpifn.org.uk/imap/). One way that you can do this is to ensure the mother gets useful guidance regarding being dairy-free both for herself and for her infant, once family foods are introduced, via referral to a paediatric dietician at the point of diagnosis (there are often long waiting lists). You may wish to read the GPIFN article that links to a number of resources for supporting parents with a child with a cows' milk allergy (Lovis, 2019). Some mothers find the site www.dylanandme.com useful in providing top tips on being dairy-free as a breastfeeding mother. First Steps Nutrition website (pharma-free!) (www.firststepsnutrition.org/) has a useful section on vegan diets for the under-5s which may be a useful resource. The app Food Maestro was developed at Guys' and St Thomas' Trust and is a useful aid to identifying foods in supermarkets and when eating out.

Back to the importance of language: simply supporting a mother in her choice to breastfeed and in encouraging her that it is entirely feasible on a dairy-free diet can make a real difference to her and her baby. Often women report that well-meaning family members or friends suggest she should stop breastfeeding as 'it's too much' to continue breastfeeding whilst dairy-free. It is only too much if the mother herself feels it is too much, ideally after she has been made aware of all the information and practical advice she needs to help it work for her.

It has been identified that infant feeding issues can represent an unmet educational need for GPs and primary care staff (Renfrew 2006). Little time on it is often spent in both undergraduate and specialist training curricula. This means that you can make a huge impact by arranging infant feeding education for GPs or trainees and primary care staff in your locality. Norwich Clinical Commissioning Group (CCG) has invested in this training and has an excellent GP Champion in Infant Feeding scheme, and at the time of writing, Surrey Heartlands ICS are also rolling out a similar programme. Practices each have an infant feeding lead who attends training in infant feeding and then disseminates this learning throughout the practice. The practice also is then awarded breastfeeding-friendly status. Such a scheme is easily replicated across other areas. It is worth coordinating funding bids with Public Health England as improving breastfeeding rates for the UK is an important public health priority. When educating clinicians I find it useful to have a GP champion co-presenting with an infant feeding advisor as it helps to have a prescriber's input and the perspective of a clinician in primary care.

There are many very useful resources available for GPs to help you to give evidence-based guidance. The GP Infant Feeding Network is a national network of GPs with an interest in infant feeding. The website www.gpifn.org.uk covers many infant feeding queries that present in primary care and has links to other useful resources for GPs. You may wish to consider developing or importing an infant feeding template for your IT system. For example, I use EMIS Web and have developed a template to support decision making for colleagues in caring for breastfeeding women and their children. The template includes tabs for the common infant feeding issues that present to primary care (mastitis, 'reflux', 'cows' milk allergy', 'poor milk supply', 'tongue tie') and links to guidance for these topics as well as to guidance for prescribing in breastfeeding. Interventions like this can help the clinicians in your practice offer evidence-based advice and support even if they have very little experience of breastfeeding or training on the topic. Including local information resources on the template can particularly help locum staff who might not know where the nearest breastfeeding clinic is.

In summary, you are in a wonderful position as a GP to change a mother's experience of breastfeeding from the moment she contacts the surgery and enters the building to the consultation and beyond. Interventions can be cheap and quick wins. Knowledge is power and by helping mothers to breastfeed for as long as they wish you can be part of improving rates of breastfeeding in this country and making a huge financial saving for the NHS, saving time for your colleagues in primary care. Most importantly, you can improve real health outcomes for children and their mothers.

References

Bolling K, Grant C, Hamlyn B, Thornton A (2005) Infant Feeding Survey 2005. Office of National Statistics 2007 (www.ic.nhs.uk/pubs/ifs2005).

Lovis M-T (2019) Cows' Milk Allergy. GP Infant Feeding Network (https://gpifn.org.uk/cma/).

Pokhrel S, Quigley MA, Fox-Rushby J, McCormick F, Williams A, Trueman P, Dodds R, Renfrew MJ (2015) Potential economic impacts from improving breastfeeding rates in the UK. *Arch Dis Child* 100(4):334–40.

Renfrew MJ, McFadden A, Dykes F, Wallace LM, Abbott S, Burt S, Anderson JK (2006) Addressing the learning deficit in breastfeeding: strategies for change. *Matern Child Nutr* 2(4):239–44.

2 Why breastfeeding matters

Natalie Shenker

A PICU consultant was musing one day about approaching her hospital board for funding to supply a targeted gut immunotherapy to patients under her care. The therapy in question had powerful antiviral, antibacterial and antifungal properties, possible antitumour activity, and a cocktail of thousands of bioactive molecules, which were readily absorbed with systemic effects on both the short- and long-term development of every organ system. And as a special bonus, the therapy was designed to be specific to the individual baby, according to that baby's genetic make-up and environment.

The consultant stopped and laughed, 'But they would never fund a lactation consultant'.

Breastfeeding matters. It isn't always a popular or easy thing to say, as we live in a culture that at best sees infant formula as biochemically equivalent to human milk, and at worst sees positive messaging around lactation as a profound threat to maternal choice and mental health. However, if we can understand better why mothers produce milk, and what it contains, supporting women to breastfeed will surely become a top public health priority.

As doctors, we pledge to uphold health and treat disease using the best available evidence. The problem is, many of our perceptions around infant feeding are based on beliefs that permeate our culture, which are absorbed over a lifetime, and our culture has had a problem with breastfeeding for decades. Therefore, very little time is spent in medical schools on teaching the normal anatomy, physiology and function of the breast, while training on breast pathology usually relates to breast lumps and cancer, rather than diagnosing and managing disorders of lactogenesis. Evidence around infant feeding practices has been diluted by decades of formula industry-sponsored studies, medical societies and training, introducing conflicts of interest that exist to reinforce the perceived equivalency between human milk and formula (Brown 2018).

More than 90% of mothers want to breastfeed their babies if asked during pregnancy. In the UK, more than 50% have given formula by the time their babies are 6 weeks, and only one in 200 will be breastfeeding by the time their baby is 1 year. More than nine out of ten mothers stop breastfeeding before they would have wished (NHS 2018).

As doctors, we have a critical role in influencing behaviour, signposting mothers. and supporting them. This book aims to be your guide to supporting mothers. Along the way, please consider challenging your inner assumptions, which may depend on somehow accepting that your own journey as a parent was failed by the society in which we live. We must challenge assumptions to ensure that the next generation of mothers are not failed in this way.

Assumption 1

Assess the available data against the premises on which they are based – these are probably wrong

Western society has viewed infant feeding through a distorted prism for almost a century, if not longer. Most people living in Western countries, including healthcare professionals, will look aghast at the concept of a baby being breastfed for more than 6 months. But when comparative biologists look at other primate species, and when tribes that have been uninfluenced by marketing or other influences of Western society are studied, something unexpected is observed. The natural term of breastfeeding can last for over 2 years and is likely to range from 4 to 7 years. In other words, this is what babies have evolved to 'expect', and what women's bodies are designed for. Recent prospective studies have started to show differences in the development of the gut microbiome and brain development between babies who are exclusively fed with human milk and those supplemented with formula, with strong dose-dependent effects (Forbes et al. 2018; Stanislawski et al. 2018).

And then we look at the trials. How can any conclusions be made in terms of long-term outcomes between trial groups where a breastfed child counts as one that has been breastfed for the first 6 weeks? How can we judge differences between groups that are 'exclusively breastfed', when we find that most of these babies received some formula in the first week (Flaherman et al. 2019)? And what can we conclude from retrospective studies where mothers are asked how they fed their babies, and how many formula feeds they gave them in the first month, several years or decades down the line?

The truth is, almost no studies exist that will tell the whole truth about the impact of our comparatively modern approach of limited-duration breastfeeding. Almost any trial on breastfeeding can be viewed with a hefty dose of scepticism because they are based on assumptions that don't mirror our evolution, that don't consider how the system was set up to function. If we consider the following statements, trials may be set up very differently:

1. Human babies expect to be fed by their mothers for 4–7 years (Dettwyler 1995; Jakobsen et al. 1996).
2. The infant gut microbiome is introduced and nourished by breastmilk (Kundu et al. 2017).
3. The gut's function in the first few months of life is not just the absorption of nutrients, but the vanguard of training of an immunocompromised neonate from environmental pathogens, supported by a multitude of components in maternal milk (oligosaccharides, lactoferrin, lysozyme, macrophages, antibodies of multiple classes and non-pathogenic microbes).
4. The gut–brain axis is now seen to be critical in determining mood states, cognition and even the basis for certain neurological diseases, including Parkinson's disease, and the role of infant feeding is critical in establishing a healthy, diverse microbiome (Fung et al. 2017).

5. The infant gut is up to 3 metres long by 40 weeks' gestation (Weaver et al. 1991), which presumably allows some redundancy if exclusive breastfeeding isn't possible, and could explain the dose and duration-dependent effects seen with exposure to formula.

Good trial data are starting to emerge, and doctors and scientists are starting to take notice of what they show. In the absence of being able to randomise babies to different methods of infant feeding, the gold-standard epidemiological approach is a large, prospective cohort study, and the first of these that specifically looked at infant feeding has been publishing results for the last few years.

However, prospective, well-controlled large cohorts such as the CHILD study are starting to show the reality, which is that any formula causes some physiological changes in the development of babies (Moossavi et al. 2019). At this stage, I need to declare that 7 and 5 years ago I freely gave both my girls significant volumes of formula in their early weeks and months and I have had to wrap my head firmly around this data. The Unicef Baby Friendly Initiative of 'when you know better, you do better' has to apply in the interests of preserving sanity. There is a dose-dependent effect, so the changes are more marked in babies who receive higher volumes of formula (microbiome changes primarily, but potentially also epigenetic changes). So far the cohort has produced data from over 2,500 children showing increased exposure to formula increases the risk of overweight at 1 year, risk of asthma and increased severity of asthma. This cohort is still young, but follow-up studies show from this rich resource and similar cohorts will be watched with interest.

Assumption 2

Formula has been designed to be as close to human milk as possible

As a biofluid, milk is vastly complex and goes far beyond nutrition. As humans, we are mammals – united almost uniquely with other mammalian species through the physiological process of lactation (the word *mamma* is Latin for breast, or duct). Diverse though the reproductive strategies of mammals are (eggs of monotremes like the duck-billed platypus, pouches of kangaroos and placentas of everything else, including humans), all mammals share lactation as the key strategy to nurture and nourish their young. Humans are the only species that has co-opted the milk of other species (e.g. cows, goats) and this has only been made viable since the invention of infant formula using pasteurised milk in the late 1800s.

The first milks developed around 250 million years ago, most likely as an evolutionary selection for mothers who could produce a fluid from their ventral surfaces to hydrate their eggs in an arid environment. If there was also passive transfer of immune-protective factors through that fluid, then those developing eggs had a selective advantage against harmful pathogens. Over time, postnatal suckling developed and mammals developed nipples along the so-called milk line. Even now, after millennia of humans just having two breasts, children of either sex being born with an additional nipple along the ventral chest or abdominal wall is not uncommon.

The point of knowing how milk evolved is that nutrition was not the primary purpose. It was hydration, and immune protection. Nutrition came later. As a tool for developing the immune system though, human milk covers all bases.

Babies are born in a relatively immunocompromised Th2 state, which means they are still reliant on maternal immunoglobulins transferred via the placenta, and whatever they ingest for immune protection (Zhang et al. 2017). Babies are born into the most lethal of environments – faeces and blood – and must rapidly tool up to combat the intense range of pathogens they will encounter. Maternal milk carries antibodies – IgA, IgG and IgM – which carry immediate immunity, along with the high maternal macrophage content of colostrum.

In the earliest days postnatally, the gut epithelium in the neonatal small bowel is relatively 'leaky'. The lack of patency between gut epithelial cells serves two purposes – to allow large molecules, such as maternal antibodies, and cells (stem cells, macrophages, etc.) in milk. Maternal stem cells from breastmilk have been found in distant organs in the baby (Molès et al. 2018). But crucially, it allows two-way communication. In the perifollicular zone of the neonate, just below the gut basement membrane, follicles packed full of naïve B cells are waiting to be told what to do. Neonatal dendritic cells sitting just beneath the gut epithelium poke tendrils out into the lumen of the gut, 'sensing' the bacteria that are starting to teem (Zhang et al. 2016). It appears that this sensing, where the dendritic cells ingest and then present bacterial antigen to the waiting naïve cells, helps to train the immune system to recognise friend from foe, patterning the B-cell and T-cell response, complement system activation and many other aspects of our complex immunity.

While we now know that babies are not born with completely sterile intestines, most of the gut microbiome is seeded postnatally. While the mode of birth and use of antibiotics perinatally can affect the microbiome pattern, the dominant exposure that determines the development of a healthy, diverse and Gram-positive (*Lactobacillus/Bifidobacterium*)-dominant microbiome is whether the baby is fed with human milk (Stewart 2018). A healthy infant gut microbiome can look very different to that of a baby fed with formula, where Gram-negative species such as *Clostridium* dominate (Baumann-Dudenhoeffer et al. 2018; Gaufin et al. 2018). Babies who have been fed with minimal even volumes of formula within the first week of birth have a microbiome that differs from an exclusively breastfed baby's microbiome (Mueller et al. 2015; Robertson et al. 2019). And we are starting to understand the associations between microbiome profiles in infancy and disease risk, including diseases as diverse as asthma (Klopp et al. 2017), obesity (Azad et al. 2018; Forbes et al. 2018), acute lymphoblastic leukaemia (Greaves 2018) and type 1 diabetes (Vatanen et al. 2018).

But nutrition is also important – babies have got to grow. Parents watch nervously as growth charts are plotted, as centiles are crossed, and mothers doubt themselves even more if the growth starts tailing off. In some babies, this is clearly pathological – severe reflux, pyloric stenosis, severe tongue tie – but in most, obsessing about growth will simply make a mother more stressed and impact her ability to lactate more.

So what nutrition is in milk? We could start talking about all the different proteins (nearly 1,000 on the latest proteome studies, of which 34 are unique to humans), fats (thousands of metabolites) and sugars (hundreds), but you would rapidly glaze over. The critical point is, yes, there are calories in milk, but almost every component has more than one function. The book *Milk* (Power and Schulkin 2016) goes into detail about how hooded seals have milk with more than 50% fat, but human breasts have a few tricks up their own sleeves. Milk changes throughout the day, the month and the years as babies develop. It responds to the needs of the babies and contains thousands of hidden functions. How many of us have heard of beta-casein, a protein that the baby can metabolise to beta-casomorphins? Beta-casomorphins act as painkillers, working on the same pain receptors as morphine. They also help nerves to develop in the brain and elsewhere (Jarmołowska et al. 2007). Human mothers are really good at extracting fats from their diet to put into milk. These fats are critical for brain and neural development.

In 2019 a group published on alkylglycerol-type ether lipids (AKGs), which are not found in infant formula or adult diets (Yu et al. 2019). AKGs are broken down by immune cells in the fatty tissue of babies and young children into platelet-activating factor, which activates IL-6/STAT3 signalling in fat cells and triggers beige adipose tissue cells to develop. Beige adipose tissue is thermogenic, creating heat by using vast amounts of energy (300 times that produced by fat-storing white adipose tissue). Once babies stop receiving AKGs, their beige fat cells transition into white adipose tissue, possibly adding another reason why formula-fed babies have a higher risk of being overweight at 1 year (Forbes et al. 2018). Taurine helps to form membranes around and inside the cell and speeds up how quickly nerve signals can be transmitted. Plasmologens help the rapid myelination of nerve fibres, which rapidly develop over the first few years of life. And leptin, a hormone, helps to suppress the appetite and may help to develop brain responses to being full, meaning that food intake is reduced over a lifetime. Lutein is essential for normal brain and eye development (Gossage et al. 2002; Jeon et al. 2018) and increases in concentration over at least the first year of lactation (the concept of milk becoming less 'nutritious' over time is the opposite of the truth: Perrin et al. 2017). There are thousands more bioactive lipids in human milk – imagine if we knew what their roles were, how staggering that realisation might be?

Lactose, the second highest constituent in human milk after water, is the main nutritional sugar. It is a disaccharide, made up of glucose and galactose – a clever quirk of evolution that allows double the amount of potential metabolisable energy to be wrapped up in the same volume of water as a glucose disaccharide alone. Basically, babies don't have to drink vast volumes to get a decent dose of readily produced energy. Lactose is responsible for how much water is in milk. It creates an osmotic gradient in the Golgi apparatus of breast epithelial cells,[1] drawing water into the Golgi and then into the milk. When lactation is not being stimulated by an infant suckling regularly, breast epithelial cells start to apoptose gradually, reducing lactose production and therefore the osmotic gradient, making milk more concentrated for fat and protein as the infant grows older (Perrin et al. 2017). This means that the developing toddler gets a higher dose of antimicrobial factors, fat and protein, with reduced levels of water and lactose.

Human milk oligosaccharides (HMOs), modified lactose and oligosaccharides are likely to be older evolutionarily than lactose and some oligosaccharides were probably busy washing over those pre-placental mammalian eggs in the desert. They are remarkable – over 200 different types of HMO have been described (Bode 2012), and at least 20 cannot be metabolised by the infant. They are there to feed the *Bifidobacterium* and *Lactobacillus* spp. that broadly constitute a health infant gut microbiome and play significant roles in supporting the developing immune system (Ruiz et al. 2017). Their functions range from prebiotics to antibacterial agents (they encapsulate pathogens, and stop them binding to the gut epithelium), contribute to the osmotic gradient, play roles in cell-to-cell communication and block adhesion sites for pathogens to enter cells. Every woman produces a slightly different HMO profile, which seems to be influenced by her genetics, environment and the genetics of the baby. The science around HMOs is developing, but it is inconceivable that supplementing infant formulas with one, two or three different types of HMO will replicate their function in human milk, and there may be associated harms.

Assumption 3

Formula has fewer 'ingredients' than human milk

If you pick up a tin of infant formula, it will list about 40 components, required to be there by law. Several tools have been developed to show how many more Lego pieces are found in breastmilk than formula. But this is missing the complexity – there are hundreds of different proteins in breastmilk, and hundreds in cows' milk. The point is that they are different: biochemically, relative concentrations and how they are metabolised. Figure 2.1 nicely shows this, using principal component analysis to look at milk samples from mothers of babies with different ages compared to three different brands of formula. The same analyses will be true for sugars, proteins, genetic signalling molecules and cell content. Milk is complex regardless of the species, but it is tailored for the specific needs of that species.

Although lists can be exhaustive, there is no doubt that the complexity of breastmilk is not just the sum of its parts, but the inter-relationship between each constituent influenced by the needs of the child and the environment of the mother. Not every component is even known, and not every one of the molecules that is known is understood, let alone their function in the unique environment of a mother's microbiome, metabolome and epigenome. The baby changes how the breast ducts work during suckling – the vacuum created allows a small amount of saliva to be sucked back into

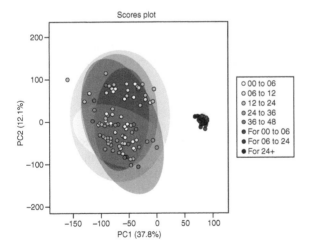

Figure 2.1 Principal component analysis (PCA) of human milk and bovine-derived commercially available ready-made formula milk for three age ranges. Clear separation is seen between human milk and formula using rapid evaporative ionisation mass spectrometry (REIMS) modalities

the breast ducts, carrying messenger molecules called microRNAs. Exactly how these molecules work in the breast to alter the composition of the milk is still not known but gives a tantalising glance at how the baby may influence the mother before s/he can even talk.

Health outcomes for babies

So where does this leave us in interpreting health outcomes for babies? Modelling of different illnesses based on the best available evidence showed that five health outcomes were incontrovertibly linked to a baby not being breastfed: necrotising enterocolitis, ear infections, bronchiolitis, gastroenteritis, maternal breast cancer. The economic burden on the NHS for the care of mothers and babies with these conditions amounted in 2012 to £40 million (Renfrew et al. 2012).

However, the model also considered that 41 diseases were likely to be linked to breastfeeding, but studies of enough quality to confirm or refute the links had not been done. Beyond that, there was a biological plausibility for more than 250 other conditions, but the research links were even weaker (Renfrew 2012). All these studies are likely to be confounded by the fact that the infant gut appears to respond to even a few doses of formula. There are likely to be few babies in the Western world who did not receive at least small volumes of infant formula or other non-human milk in the first few days and weeks of life. In the UK, around 20% of babies do not receive colostrum. Although the UK Infant Feeding Survey was stopped after the 2010 results were published, giving no data on rates across the country, some evidence suggests that more than 50% of mothers stop feeding within the first week of their baby's life (Cleminson et al. 2015; Victora et al. 2016).

The economic costs of not breastfeeding have recently been estimated at US$1 billion each day globally (Rollins et al. 2016; Walters et al. 2019). When you consider milk as a whole-body developmental tool, underpinning immune system, neurological and gut development in addition to other organ systems (heart, eye, lungs, skin, muscle, lungs), the enormity of not being fed with mother's milk starts to sink in. Modern epidemics of Western lifestyle – heart disease, obesity, hypertension, diabetes – could start to make a little more sense.

Maternal health

From a purely evolutionary perspective, having babies is the most critical role of a female human – perpetuating her genetic code. Before modern medicine, successful lactation would have been the lifeline for infants. It would make little sense if mothers did not gain an advantage from this process, given the relative constraints on her for the metabolic load required to lactate (lactating breasts are estimated to consume more energy than brain tissue). Breasts are primary immune organs, although rarely categorised as such in anatomy or physiology textbooks, and the production of immune cells and antibodies presumably enhances maternal immunity at a period when she may be relatively vulnerable postnatally, as well as infant immunity. Both mother and baby need to benefit from lactation to survive evolutionary pressures.

Again, much of the research in the area of maternal health (and there isn't a great deal) is confounded by incorrect assumptions, as described at the start of this chapter. For example, almost 20 years ago, a large *Lancet* meta-analysis showed that, of all risk factors considered, breastfeeding didn't play much of a role in off-setting a woman's risk of ductal breast cancer – a yearly reduction in risk of 4.3% over a lifetime (Collaborative Group on Hormonal Factors in Breast Cancer 2002). When I was in surgical training, we learned that age, genetic susceptibility and hormonal factors were much more important. Then things changed – breast cancer was classified a few years later into five discrete pathological subtypes, characterised by a different cell type of origin in the breast ductal tissue. A few years later, when enough studies had been done looking at epidemiological risk factors for the different subtypes, meta-analyses showed the startling result that breastfeeding was highly protective of the most aggressive subtype of breast cancer, triple-negative disease (Islami et al. 2015; Lambertini et al. 2016). This form of cancer tends to affect younger women, those who develop cancer during pregnancy and those with a *BRCA1* mutation. A further meta-analysis showed that breastfeeding was associated with risk reductions of over 50% for breast cancer in women who were *BRCA1* carriers (Jernstrom et al. 2004; Pan et al. 2014), suggesting a fascinating insight into the biology of this disease, and potential strategies for prevention and treatment, specifically around maximising the chance of breastfeeding. Intriguingly, breastfeeding in women with a *BRCA1* mutation also reduces their risk of ovarian cancer (Kotsopoulos et al. 2015). Often though, women who carry a *BRCA1* mutation and become pregnant are advised not to breast-feed, so it is easier to assess for tumour growth shortly after the birth. Smaller studies have shown similar protective effects against forms of ovarian cancer (Gaitskell et al. 2018) and endometrial cancer (Jordan et al. 2017; Ma et al. 2018), as well as, intriguingly, oesophageal cancer (Zhu et al. 2017). Which brings us back to the role of the breast as a primary immune organ, and the tantalising prospect that immune surveillance against tumours acts systemically during the period of lactation.

Beyond cancer, mothers appear to benefit from feeding in a multitude of physiological and psychological ways, with duration-dependent protective effects apparent for cardiovascular disease (Schwarz et al. 2009; Nguyen et al. 2017), type 2 diabetes (Chowdhury et al. 2015; Gunderson et al. 2018), hypertension (Stuebe et al. 2011), stroke (Jacobson et al. 2018), multiple sclerosis (Hellwig et al. 2015 (relapses); Langer-Gould et al. 2017 (onset)), rheumatoid arthritis (Chen et al. 2015), endometriosis (Farland et al. 2017) and postnatal depression (Brown et al. 2016; Chaput et al. 2016).

Science, whether basic mechanistic studies of single human milk components, or global health studies into the impacts on infant health and maternal mental and physical health, has overwhelmingly changed the conversation around infant feeding in recent years. Mothers matter. Most want to breastfeed their babies, and the majority will be physiologically able to do so if given the right information and support antenatally and in the early hours and days postnatally. There are wonders in breastfeeding, but as with any biological system, sometimes it fails, sometimes mothers are ill or die and sometimes it just doesn't develop properly. This book will take you through the management of each of these settings, but overwhelmingly, most mothers will be able to fulfil their fundamental evolutionary drive to nourish their baby.

There are perhaps few interventions in the role of a medic that can have such a major impact in the short and long term on both child and mother, family and society, as supporting a mother to establish and maintain her milk supply. This book aims to give a clear pathway for when and how medics should walk alongside expectant and new mothers to support and comfort them, signposting to support services and training in these skills ourselves, and crucially always treating them with compassion at what can be the most vulnerable of times. You can literally change a family's future with some relatively simple knowledge and signposting.

> In all mammalian species the reproductive cycle comprises both pregnancy and breast-feeding: in the absence of latter, none of these species, man included, could have survived.
>
> (Dr Bo Vahlquist, Paediatrician, 1981)

Note

1 A single-cell layer that lines the milk ducts, of which some differentiate into lactocytes during pregnancy. The breast is the only organ that terminally differentiates during pregnancy, although recent functional MRI studies suggest that the maternal brain could also be classed as such (Hoekzema et al. 2017)!

References

Academy of Breastfeeding Medicine (2012) ABM affirms breastfeeding beyond infancy as the biological norm [Press release]. https://bfmed.wordpress.com/2012/05/15/abm-affirms-breastfeeding-beyond-infancy-as-the-biological-norm

Azad MB, Vehling L, Chan D, Klopp A, Nickel NC, McGavock JM, Becker AB, Mandhane PJ, Turvey SE, Moraes TJ, Taylor MS, Lefebvre DL, Sears MR, Subbarao P; CHILD Study Investigators (2018). Infant feeding and weight gain: separating breast milk from breastfeeding and formula from food. *Pediatrics* 142(4).

Baumann-Dudenhoeffer AM, D'Souza AW, Tarr PI, Warner BB, Dantas G (2018) Infant diet and maternal gestational weight gain predict early metabolic maturation of gut microbiomes. *Nat Med* 24(12):1822–9.

Bode L (2012) Human milk oligosaccharides: every baby needs a sugar mama. *Glycobiology* 22(9):1147–62.

Brown A (2018) Dispatches: Breastfeeding Uncovered [Television programme], 27 July. www.imdb.com/title/tt8717290/

Brown A, Rance J, Bennett P (2016) Understanding the relationship between breastfeeding and postnatal depression: the role of pain and physical difficulties. *J Adv Nurs* 72(2):273–82.

Chaput KH, Nettel-Aguirre A, Musto R, Adair CE, Tough SC (2016) Breastfeeding difficulties and supports and risk of postpartum depression in a cohort of women who have given birth in Calgary: a prospective cohort study. *CMAJ Open* 4(1):E103–9.

Chen H, Wang J, Zhou W, Yin H, Wang M (2015) Breastfeeding and risk of rheumatoid arthritis: a systematic review and metaanalysis. *J Rheumatol* 42(9):1563–9.

Chowdhury R, Sinha B, Sankar MJ, Taneja S, Bhandari N, Rollins N, Bahl R, Martines J (2015) Breastfeeding and maternal health outcomes: a systematic review and meta-analysis. *Acta Paediatr* 104(467):96–113.

Cleminson J, Oddie S, Renfrew MJ, McGuire W (2015) Being baby friendly: evidence-based breastfeeding support. *Arch Dis Child Fetal Neonatal Ed* 100(2):F173–8.

Collaborative Group on Hormonal Factors in Breast Cancer (2002) Breast cancer and breastfeeding: collaborative reanalysis of individual data from 47 epidemiological studies in 30 countries, including 50302 women with breast cancer and 96973 women without the disease. *Lancet* 20;360(9328):187–95.

Dettwyler KA (1995) A time to wean. In: Stuart-Macadam P, Dettwyler KA (eds) *Breastfeeding: Biocultural Perspectives*. Aldine Trasaction.

Farland LV, Eliassen AH, Tamimi RM, Spiegelman D, Michels KB, Missmer SA (2017) History of breast feeding and risk of incident endometriosis: prospective cohort study. *BMJ* 358:j3778.

Flaherman VJ, Cabana MD, McCulloch CE, Paul IM (2019) Effect of early limited formula on breastfeeding duration in the first year of life: a randomized clinical trial. *JAMA Pediatr* 1;173(8):729–35.

Forbes JD, Azad MB, Vehling L, Tun HM, Konya TB, Guttman DS, Field CJ, Lefebvre D, Sears MR, Becker AB, Mandhane PJ, Turvey SE, Moraes TJ, Subbarao P, Scott JA, Kozyrskyj AL; Canadian Healthy Infant Longitudinal Development (CHILD) Study Investigators (2018). Association of exposure to formula in the hospital and subsequent infant feeding practices with gut microbiota and risk of overweight in the first year of life. *JAMA Pediatr* 172(7):e181161.

Fung TC, Olson CA, Hsiao EY (2017) Interactions between the microbiota, immune and nervous systems in health and disease. *Nat Neurosci* 20(2):145–55. doi: 10.1038/nn.4476.

Gaitskell K, Green J, Pirie K, Barnes I, Hermon C, Reeves GK, Beral V; Million Women Study Collaborators (2018). Histological subtypes of ovarian cancer associated with parity and breastfeeding in the prospective Million Women Study. *Int J Cancer* 142(2):281–9.

Gaufin T, Tobin NH, Aldrovandi GM (2018) The importance of the microbiome in pediatrics and pediatric infectious diseases. *Curr Opin Pediatr* 30(1):117–24.

Gossage CP, Deyhim M, Yamini S, Douglass LW, Moser-Veillon PB (2002) Carotenoid composition of human milk during the first month postpartum and the response to beta-carotene supplementation. *Am J Clin Nutr* 76(1):193–7.

Greaves M (2018) A causal mechanism for childhood acute lymphoblastic leukaemia. *Nat Rev Cancer* 18(8):471–84.

Gunderson EP, Lewis CE, Lin Y, Sorel M, Gross M, Sidney S, Jacobs DR Jr, Shikany JM, Quesenberry CP Jr (2018) Lactation duration and progression to diabetes in women across the childbearing years: the 30-year CARDIA study. *JAMA Intern Med* 178(3):328–37.

Hellwig K, Rockhoff M, Herbstritt S, Borisow N, Haghikia A, Elias-Hamp B, Menck S, Gold R, Langer-Gould A (2015) Exclusive breastfeeding and the effect on postpartum multiple sclerosis relapses. *JAMA Neurol* 72(10):1132–8.

Hoekzema E, Barba-Müller E, Pozzobon C, Picado M, Lucco F, García-García D, Soliva JC, Tobeña A, Desco M, Crone EA, Ballesteros A, Carmona S, Vilarroya O (2017) Pregnancy leads to long-lasting changes in human brain structure. *Nat Neurosci* 20(2):287–96.

Islami F, Liu Y, Jemal A, Zhou J, Weiderpass E, Colditz G, Boffetta P, Weiss M (2015) Breastfeeding and breast cancer risk by receptor status – a systematic review and meta-analysis. *Ann Oncol* 26(12):2398–407.

Jacobson LT, Hade EM, Collins TC, Margolis KL, Waring ME, Van Horn LV, Silver B, Sattari M, Bird CE, Kimminau K, Wambach K, Stefanick ML (2018) Breastfeeding history and risk of stroke among parous postmenopausal women in the Women's Health Initiative. *J Am Heart Assoc* 7(17):e008739.

Jakobsen MS, Sodemann M, Molbak K, Aacy P (1996) Reason for termination of breastfeeding and the length of breastfeeding. *Int J Epidemiol* 25(1):115–21.

Jarmołowska B, Sidor K, Iwan M, Bielikowicz K, Kaczmarski M, Kostyra E, Kostyra H (2007) Changes of beta-casomorphin content in human milk during lactation. *Peptides* 28(10):1982–6.

Jeon S, Ranard KM, Neuringer M, Johnson EE, Renner L, Kuchan MJ, Pereira SL, Johnson EJ, Erdman JW Jr (2018) Lutein is differentially deposited across brain regions following formula or breast feeding of infant rhesus macaques. *J Nutr* 148(1):31–9.

Jernström H, Lubinski J, Lynch HT, Ghadirian P, Neuhausen S, Isaacs C, Weber BL, Horsman D, Rosen B, Foulkes WD, Friedman E, Gershoni-Baruch R, Ainsworth P, Daly M, Garber J, Olsson H, Sun P, Narod SA (2004) Breast-feeding and the risk of breast cancer in BRCA1 and BRCA2 mutation carriers. *J Natl Cancer Inst* 96(14):1094–8.

Jordan SJ, Na R, Johnatty SE, Wise LA, Adami HO, Brinton LA, Chen C, Cook LS, Dal Maso L, De Vivo I, Freudenheim JL, Friedenreich CM, La Vecchia C, McCann SE, Moysich KB, Lu L, Olson SH, Palmer JR, Petruzella S, Pike MC, Rebbeck TR, Ricceri F, Risch HA, Sacerdote

C, Setiawan VW, Sponholtz TR, Shu XO, Spurdle AB, Weiderpass E, Wentzensen N, Yang HP, Yu H, Webb PM (2017) Breastfeeding and endometrial cancer risk: an analysis from the Epidemiology of Endometrial Cancer Consortium. *Obstet Gynecol* 129(6):1059–67.

Klopp A, Vehling L, Becker AB, Subbarao P, Mandhane PJ, Turvey SE, Lefebvre DL, Sears MR; CHILD Study Investigators (2017). Modes of infant feeding and the risk of childhood asthma: a prospective birth cohort study. *J Pediatr* 190:192–9.e2.

Kotsopoulos J, Lubinski J, Gronwald J, Cybulski C, Demsky R, Neuhausen SL, Kim-Sing C, Tung N, Friedman S, Senter L, Weitzel J, Karlan B, Moller P, Sun P, Narod SA; Hereditary Breast Cancer Clinical Study Group (2015). Factors influencing ovulation and the risk of ovarian cancer in BRCA1 and BRCA2 mutation carriers. *Int J Cancer* 137(5):1136–46.

Kundu P, Blacher E, Elinav E, Pettersson S (2017) Our gut microbiome: the evolving inner self. *Cell* 171(7):1481–93.

Lambertini M, Santoro L, Del Mastro L, Nguyen B, Livraghi L, Ugolini D, Peccatori FA, Azim HA Jr (2016) Reproductive behaviors and risk of developing breast cancer according to tumor subtype: a systematic review and meta-analysis of epidemiological studies. *Cancer Treat Rev* 49:65–76.

Langer-Gould A, Smith JB, Hellwig K, Gonzales E, Haraszti S, Koebnick C, Xiang A (2017) Breastfeeding, ovulatory years, and risk of multiple sclerosis. *Neurology* 89(6):563–9.

Ma X, Zhao LG, Sun JW, Yang Y, Zheng JL, Gao J, Xiang YB (2018) Association between breastfeeding and risk of endometrial cancer: a meta-analysis of epidemiological studies. *Eur J Cancer Prev* 27(2):144–51.

Molès JP, Tuaillon E, Kankasa C, Bedin AS, Nagot N, Marchant A, McDermid JM, Van de Perre P (2018) Breastmilk cell trafficking induces microchimerism-mediated immune system maturation in the infant. *Pediatr Allergy Immunol* 29(2):133–43.

Moossavi S, Sepehri S, Robertson B, Bode L, Goruk S, Field CJ, Lix LM, de Souza RJ, Becker AB, Mandhane PJ, Turvey SE, Subbarao P, Moraes TJ, Lefebvre DL, Sears MR, Khafipour E, Azad MB (2019) Composition and variation of the human milk microbiota are influenced by maternal and early-life factors. *Cell Host Microbe* 25(2):324–35.e4

Mueller NT, Bakacs E, Combellick J, Grigoryan Z, Dominguez-Bello MG (2015) The infant microbiome development: mom matters. *Trends Mol Med* 21(2):109–17.

Nguyen B, Jin K, Ding D (2017) Breastfeeding and maternal cardiovascular risk factors and outcomes: a systematic review. *PLoS One* 12(11):e0187923.

NHS (2018) National Maternity Review. www.england.nhs.uk/mat-transformation/implementing-better-births/mat-review/

Pan H, He Z, Ling L, Ding Q, Chen L, Zha X, Zhou W, Liu X, Wang S (2014) Reproductive factors and breast cancer risk among BRCA1 or BRCA2 mutation carriers: results from ten studies. *Cancer Epidemiol* 38(1):1–8.

Perrin MT, Fogleman AD, Newburg DS, Allen JC (2017) A longitudinal study of human milk composition in the second year postpartum: implications for human milk banking. *Matern Child Nutr* 13(1).

Power M, Schulkin J (2016). *Milk*. Baltimore, MD: Johns Hopkins University Press, p. 296.

Renfrew MJ, Pokhrel S, Quigley M, McCormick F, Fox-Rushby J, Dodds R, Duffy S, Trueman P, Williams A (2012) Preventing disease and saving resources: the potential contribution of increasing breastfeeding rates in the UK. Unicef UK.

Robertson RC, Manges AR, Finlay B, Prendergast AJ (2019) The human microbiome and child growth – first 1000 days and beyond. *Trends Microbiol* 27(2):131–47.

Rollins NC, Bhandari N, Hajeebhoy N, Horton S, Lutter CK, Martines JC, Piwoz EG, Richter LM, Victora CG; Lancet Breastfeeding Series Group (2016) Why invest, and what it will take to improve breastfeeding practices? *Lancet* 387(10017):491–504.

Ruiz L, Delgado S, Ruas-Madiedo P, Sánchez B, Margolles A (2017) Bifidobacteria and their molecular communication with the immune system. *Front Microbiol* 8:2345.

Schwarz EB, Ray RM, Stuebe AM, Allison MA, Ness RB, Freiberg MS, Cauley JA (2009) Duration of lactation and risk factors for maternal cardiovascular disease. *Obstet Gynecol* 113(5):974–82.

Stanislawski MA, Dabelea D, Wagner BD, Iszatt N, Dahl C, Sontag MK, Knight R, Lozupone CA, Eggesbo M (2018) Gut microbiota in the first 2 years of life and the association with body mass index at age 12 in a Norwegian birth cohort. *mBio* 9:e01751-18. doi:10.1128/mBio.01751-18.

Stewart CJ, Ajami NJ, O'Brien JL, Hutchinson DS, Smith DP, Wong MC, Ross MC, Lloyd RE, Doddapaneni H, Metcalf GA, Muzny D, Gibbs RA, Vatanen T, Huttenhower C, Xavier RJ, Rewers M, Hagopian W, Toppari J, Ziegler AG, She JX, Akolkar B, Lernmark A, Hyoty H, Vehik K, Krischer JP, Petrosino JF (2018) Temporal development of the gut microbiome in early childhood from the TEDDY study. *Nature* 562(7728):583–8.

Stuebe AM, Schwarz EB, Grewen K, Rich-Edwards JW, Michels KB, Foster EM, Curhan G, Forman J (2011) Duration of lactation and incidence of maternal hypertension: a longitudinal cohort study. *Am J Epidemiol* 174(10):1147–58.

Vatanen T, Franzosa EA, Schwager R, Tripathi S, Arthur TD, Vehik K, Lernmark Å, Hagopian WA, Rewers MJ, She JX, Toppari J, Ziegler AG, Akolkar B, Krischer JP, Stewart CJ, Ajami NJ, Petrosino JF, Gevers D, Lähdesmäki H, Vlamakis H, Huttenhower C, Xavier RJ (2018) The human gut microbiome in early-onset type 1 diabetes from the TEDDY study. *Nature* 562(7728):589–94.

Victora CG, Bahl R, Barros AJ, França GV, Horton S, Krasevec J, Murch S, Sankar MJ, Walker N, Rollins NC; Lancet Breastfeeding Series Group (2016) Breastfeeding in the 21st century: epidemiology, mechanisms, and lifelong effect. *Lancet* 387(10017):475–90.

Walters DD, Phan LTH, Mathisen R (2019) The cost of not breastfeeding: global results from a new tool. *Health Policy Plan* pii: czz050.

Weaver LT, Austin S, Cole TJ (1991). Small intestinal length: a factor essential for gut adaptation. *Gut* 32(11):1321–3.

Yu H, Dilbaz S, Coßmann J, Hoang AC, Diedrich V, Herwig A, Harauma A, Hoshi Y, Moriguchi T, Landgraf K, Körner A, Lucas C, Brodesser S, Balogh L, Thuróczy J, Karemore G, Kuefner MS, Park EA, Rapp C, Travers JB, Röszer T (2019) Breast milk alkylglycerols sustain beige adipocytes through adipose tissue macrophages. *J Clin Invest* 129(6):2485–99.

Zhang Z, Li J, Zheng W, Zhao G, Zhang H, Wang X, Guo 0, Qin C, Shi Y (2016) Peripheral lymphoid volume expansion and maintenance are controlled by gut microbiota via RALDH+ dendritic cells. *Immunity* 44(2):330–42.

Zhu Y, Yue D, Yuan B, Zhu L, Lu M (2017) Reproductive factors are associated with oesophageal cancer risk: results from a meta-analysis of observational studies. *Eur J Cancer Prev* 26(1):1–9.

Zhang X, Zhivaki D, Lo-Man R (2017) Unique aspects of the perinatal immune system. *Nat Rev Immunol* 17(8):495–507.

3   Why are breastfeeding rates in the UK so low?

Amy Brown

- Many women want to breastfeed but their ability to do so is affected by complex biological, psychological and cultural factors.
- Responsive feeding, i.e. feeding whenever the baby signals to be fed, is important for building milk supply. Babies will often feed every 2 hours or more.
- Absolute inability to produce any breastmilk is rare; however, many more women end up with insufficient milk supply through processes that separate them from their baby, dissuade them from feeding responsively or promote formula as a solution to normal infant behaviour.
- If women present with pain, difficulty or low milk supply discuss their wider feeding experiences. Are they feeding frequently? Have they been able to access professional support? Do they have concerns about feeding in front of others? Or worries about feeding too often?
- Understanding a woman's family history is also important. How did other people in her family feed, or how was she herself fed? Are they supportive of her breastfeeding? Are they helping or hindering her? What about her friends?
- It is normal for infants to wake frequently, feed frequently and want to be held. Moving to formula milk is unlikely to change this normal infant behaviour. If a mother needs support, suggest alternative ways others can help her other than using a bottle, e.g. preparing her meals, doing housework or holding the baby in between feeds.

Chapter 2 highlighted the issue of low breastfeeding rates in the UK but it is important to consider why these are occurring. Breastfeeding is important to many mothers (Brown 2018) but many are not able to breastfeed for as long as they hoped, putting them at increased risk of postnatal depression (Brown et al. 2016). Conversely, in other countries, including in Northern Europe and Australasia, rates are far higher (Victora et al. 2016).

Why are these issues occurring so differently between different regions? The answer lies in understanding the multiple influences on why women plan to and are able to breastfeed. Insufficient milk (perceived or otherwise) is one of the top reasons why women stop breastfeeding (McAndrew et al. 2012). Although physical factors such as structural and endocrine factors can affect women's ability to produce sufficient milk in some cases, absolute lack of milk is rare (Lawrence and Lawrence 2001). Instead, complex psychological, social and cultural factors often affect women's knowledge and behaviour which in turn can lead to low milk supply and breastfeeding difficulties (Rollins et al. 2016).

Understanding milk supply

A good milk supply is critical for breastfeeding success. Milk is produced in three main stages (Neville et al. 2001). During pregnancy (lactogenesis one) milk production will start at around 20 weeks, limited in amount by high levels of circulating progesterone. After the placenta is delivered levels of progesterone drop rapidly whilst prolactin rises (lactogenesis two). This hormonal response leads to mature milk production. However, after this stage, the amount of milk produced is driven not by the hormonal system but by how much milk is removed from the breast (lactogenesis three). Broadly, the more milk that is removed, the more is produced to replace it. If less milk is removed, milk production slows down.

Many of the complications that women experience with low milk supply can be linked back to what happens in lactogenesis stage three. If an infant is fed frequently and responsively (e.g. whenever the baby wants feeding, which is often at least every 2 hours or more) then this is associated with a greater milk supply and fewer complications. Conversely, attempting to limit feeds or feed to a strict maternal-led routine has been linked to a drop in milk supply, greater pain and difficulties and breastfeeding cessation (Brown et al. 2011b; Brown and Arnott 2014). Although not all breastfeeding challenges are linked to feeding patterns it often plays an influencing role.

This chapter presents the main reasons why women stop breastfeeding (often before they are ready) and how these factors often directly have an impact upon their milk supply.

Pain and difficulties with latch

Pain and latching difficulties are common reasons for stopping breastfeeding in the first week (McAndrew et al. 2012). Pain and nipple trauma can cause significant psychological distress and can lead to women trying to reduce feeding frequency, impacting upon milk supply (McClellan et al. 2012).

Birth complications can increase women's risk of experiencing these issues. As we will see, hormonal disruption, residual pain and separation of mother and baby can delay mature milk supply and lead to an infant who is less effective at removing milk, leading to increased pain, complications with latch and a lower milk supply (Brown et al. 2013).

Lack of professional support

At the heart of a good milk supply is an effective and comfortable latch, but often women, especially first-time mothers with little experience of seeing breastfeeding in their communities, need additional support in positioning and attachment. Breastfeeding may be natural but that does not necessarily mean it is intuitive or easy to latch an infant on, especially when your experience of feeding infants has been the positioning and sucking style of bottle-fed infants (Brown et al. 2011c).

Women benefit from expert professional support with getting breastfeeding off to the best start, yet in many overstretched hospitals staff do not have time to sit with women and give them the time and investment they need, leading to an increased likelihood of physical difficulties and pain (Hauck et al. 2011).

Poor societal understanding of normal infant behaviour

Infants are vulnerable in their early stages of development and have frequent, regular needs. The best outcomes occur when infants are cared for responsively, meeting those needs (Evans and Porter 2009). This includes frequent nighttime care (McKenna et al. 2007), feeding frequently and irregularly (Barr et al. 1991) and being held the majority of the time by a caregiver (Konner 1977; Trevathan and Trevathan 2010).

However, mothers often report that these normal behaviours can cause considerable anxiety or perceptions of needing to 'fix' the infant, exacerbated by societal messages that tell them that they should have a 'good baby' who is in a predictable routine (Arnott and Brown 2013). This can lead to mothers attempting to schedule feeds (Brown 2013) or not respond to their infant at night (Harries and Brown 2019a), which can lead to an increased risk of breastfeeding difficulties or lower milk supply (Brown et al. 2011b).

Some may believe the societal messages that breastfeeding increases the likelihood of infants waking at night, but research shows that mode of feeding typically has little impact on infant sleep (Brown and Harries 2015). Moreover, attempting to encourage an infant into a more scheduled 'routine' often doesn't work and can increase risk of postnatal depression (Harries and Brown 2019b) alongside damaging breastfeeding (Brown and Arnott 2014).

Maternal mental health

The dispersion of Western families means that many new parents have little experience or understanding of caring for a newborn (Cusk 2014). Many new mothers feel shocked, overwhelmed, even regretful of their new lives (Leigh and Milgrom 2008). The isolation of many new mothers can exacerbate this (Paris et al. 2005).

These emotions and experiences can put mothers at increased risk of postnatal depression (Henderson et al. 2003) which in turn is often associated with an increased risk of breastfeeding cessation (Brown et al. 2016). Everything feels more challenging when you are experiencing depression, and mothers may hope that stopping breastfeeding may fix this (Gonidakis et al. 2008). Others may suggest that they can help out by feeding the baby and the mother needs to rest and care for herself (Brown et al. 2011b). Unfortunately, cessation of breastfeeding can sometimes increase risk of further depression, in part due to the reduction in the protective hormones of breastfeeding such as oxytocin (Kendall-Tackett 2007), but also because breastfeeding is valuable to new mothers and can feel like something they are doing 'right' (Brown 2018).

It is also reliant on another caregiver stepping in and supporting the mother with feeding, and in many cases this support may not be regularly available. There are multiple other ways family and friends could support mothers (such as undertaking housework, making her meals or holding the baby in between feeds) that do not involve her having to stop breastfeeding.

Family attitudes

A mother's intention to initiate and continue breastfeeding can be heavily affected by the attitudes and experiences of those around her (Darwent et al. 2016). Mothers who were themselves breastfed are more likely to start and continue breastfeeding (Ekstrom et al. 2003), whilst if a woman was bottlefed, she is less likely to breastfeed (Susin et al. 2005). A grandmother who has breastfed successfully will be more able to offer both practical and emotional support (Ekstrom et al. 2003), whereas knowledge, attitudes and ability to support may be different amongst grandmothers with experience of bottlefeeding (Hoddinott and Pill 1999).

The mechanisms behind this are complex. Grandmothers who struggled themselves with breastfeeding may have negative memories that they wish to stop their daughter experiencing (Brown et al. 2011d). Those who did not breastfeed, or felt they had to do so discreetly, may feel uncomfortable with their daughter doing so in front of others or publicly (Trickey et al. 2017). New mothers really value emotional and practical support from their own mother, but if she does not have any experience (or any positive experience) of breastfeeding she may not be able to offer this or may offer outdated advice (Grassley and Eschiti 2008). Watching her daughter breastfeed may also bring back negative emotions, concerns or even jealousy (Grassley and Eschiti 2008).

Partner attitudes

A woman's partner can also affect her intention and ability to breastfeed. Broadly, if the partner is supportive, the woman is more likely to be able to continue, but if the partner does not or cannot support her, she may find breastfeeding more challenging (Swanson 2005). Although much of the research for partner support has focused on the role of fathers, it is likely that some influences can be generalised to same-sex couples – albeit with some different challenges involved (Walker 2017).

Most fathers are broadly supportive of breastfeeding, seeing it as their partner's decision (Brown and Davies 2014). However, many lack the understanding or skills that would best support their partner to breastfeed (Sheriff and Hall 2011). Some can feel excluded and worry that they are not bonding with their baby (Pontes et al. 2009). Others perceive formula as more convenient and safer (Henderson et al. 2011). Some fathers feel embarrassed at their partner breastfeeding in public (Brown and Davies 2014). All of these may interfere with a mother's ability or desire to feed her baby responsively, with fathers offering to give a bottle instead for more opportunity to bond.

Negative public attitudes

Unfortunately, despite women being protected to breastfeed their baby by law in the UK (Maternity Action UK 2018), many feel that breastfeeding is viewed negatively or have felt judged or criticised by others for feeding in public (Hoddinott et al. 2012). Somewhat unsurprisingly, if a woman feels worried about breastfeeding in public, she is less likely to do so, or even to breastfeed at all (Thomson and Dykes 2011). In the last UK infant feeding survey, just 58% of mothers had ever breastfed in public, with many who did so feeling very self-conscious and worried that they were going to be approached and told to stop. Only 8% reported that they felt comfortable breastfeeding whenever and wherever they liked (McAndrew et al. 2012).

Aside from making women feel uncomfortable in public this can have a negative impact on whether a woman continues breastfeeding. Some, fearing judgement, will decide to use formula in public which can impact on their milk supply. Others will try to time feeds around leaving the house, finding this overly complicated and restrictive (Brown et al. 2011a).

Returning to work

Returning to work is another common reason why women stop breastfeeding before they are ready (Kosmala-Anderson and Wallace 2006). Although women do have some legal rights in the UK in the workplace when breastfeeding, these often do not go far enough. These include making sure women have somewhere safe to rest, which should include a space to lie down, and doing a risk assessment to make sure that the environment is safe to work in. Further recommended guidance suggests that women should have access to a private room to express in (not a toilet) and a fridge in which to store milk (Maternity Action UK 2018).

However, many women do not have this support and are too embarrassed or anxious about asking for it (Kosmala-Anderson and Wallace 2006). Others find their employer openly hostile and are told they cannot express in the workplace (Gatrell 2007). Some women feel that colleagues think they are not capable in their role for continuing to breastfeed (Shildrick 1997), although voicing that opinion would be an offence under bullying and harassment in the workplace law (ACAS 2014).

Promotion of breastmilk substitutes

Under the World Health Organization *International Code of Marketing of Breast-Milk Substitutes*, in the UK women should not receive any promotion of such products for infants under 6 months old (WHO 1981). The reasons for this are clear. In the USA, where promotion of such products is allowed, a Cochrane review found that women who are given free samples of formula milk are less likely to continue breastfeeding (Donnelly et al. 2000). Other research has also found a negative impact of formula samples on breastfeeding duration (Rosenberg et al. 2008; Feldman-Winter et al. 2012)

Although in the UK promoting first-stage formula milk is illegal, industry gets around this legislation by promoting follow-on formula milks aimed at infants over 6 months old. Brand advertising means that this has a knock-on effect on stage one formula milk products (Park et al. 1991). Research has shown that many people mistake follow-on formula adverts for first-stage formula promotion (Berry et al. 2012) or do not realise there is any difference between the products, even believing follow-on formula milk must be more nutritious (McAndrew et al. 2012).

Breastfeeding should be a public health responsibility, creating the environment in which women are supported to feed their babies. Investment is needed across perinatal health services to give women the best possible start to motherhood and caring for their infant. Legislation protecting their rights in the workplace and public spaces must be upheld. It is not enough simply to tell women that breastfeeding is best for their babies without funding a societal level support system to enable them to do so (Brown et al. 2016).

References

ACAS (2014) *Accommodating Breastfeeding Employees in the Workplace.* London: ACAS.

Arnott B, Brown A (2013) An exploration of parenting behaviours and attitudes during early infancy: association with maternal and infant characteristics. *Infant Child Dev* 22(4):349–61.

Barr RG, Konner M, Bakeman R, Adamson L (1991) Crying in! Kung San infants: a test of the cultural specificity hypothesis. *Dev Med Child Neurol* 33(7):601–10.

Berry NJ, Jones SC, Iverson D (2012) Toddler milk advertising in Australia: infant formula advertising in disguise? *Australas Market J* 20(1):24–7.

Brown A (2017) Breastfeeding as a public health responsibility: a review of the evidence. *J Hum Nutr Diet* 30(6):759–70.

Brown A (2018) What do women lose if they are prevented from meeting their breastfeeding goals? *Clin Lactat* 9(4):200–7.

Brown A, Arnott B (2014) Breastfeeding duration and early parenting behaviour: the importance of an infant-led, responsive style. *PloS One* 9(2):e83893.

Brown A, Davies R (2014) Fathers' experiences of supporting breastfeeding: challenges for breastfeeding promotion and education. *Matern Child Nutr* 10(4):510–26.

Brown A, Harries V (2015) Infant sleep and night feeding patterns during later infancy: association with breastfeeding frequency, daytime complementary food intake, and infant weight. *Breastfeed Med* 10(5):246–52.

Brown A, Jordan S (2013) Impact of birth complications on breastfeeding duration: an internet survey. *J Adv Nurs* 69(4):828–39.

Brown A, Lee M (2013) Breastfeeding is associated with a maternal feeding style low in control from birth. *PloS One* 8(1):e54229.

Brown A, Raynor P, Lee M (2011a) Healthcare professionals' and mothers' perceptions of factors that influence decisions to breastfeed or formula feed infants: a comparative study. *J Adv Nursing* 67(9):1993–2003.

Brown A, Raynor P, Lee M (2011b) Maternal control of child-feeding during breast and formula feeding in the first 6 months post-partum. *J Hum Nutr Diet* 24(2):177–86.

Brown A, Raynor P, Lee M (2011c) Healthcare professionals' and mothers' perceptions of factors that influence decisions to breastfeed or formula feed infants: a comparative study. J *Adv Nurs* 67(9):1993–2003.

Brown A, Raynor P, Lee M (2011d) Young mothers who choose to breast feed: the importance of being part of a supportive breast-feeding community. Midwifery 27(1): 53–9.

Brown A, Rance J, Bennett P (2016) Understanding the relationship between breastfeeding and postnatal depression: the role of pain and physical difficulties. *J Adv Nurs* 72(2):273–82.

Cusk R (2014) *A Life's Work.* Faber & Faber.

Darwent KL, McInnes RJ, Swanson V (2016) The Infant Feeding Genogram: a tool for exploring family infant feeding history and identifying support needs. *BMC Pregnancy Childbirth* 16(1):315.

Donnelly A, Snowden HH, Renfrew MJ (2000) Commercial hospital discharge packs for breastfeeding women. *Cochrane Database System Rev* (2).

Ekström A, Widström AM, Nissen E (2003) Breastfeeding support from partners and grandmothers: perceptions of Swedish women. *Birth* 30(4):261–6.

Evans CA, Porter CL (2009) The emergence of mother–infant co-regulation during the first year: links to infants' developmental status and attachment. *Infant Behav Dev* 32(2):147–58.

Feldman-Winter L, Grossman X, Palaniappan A (2012) Removal of industry-sponsored formula sample packs from the hospital: does it make a difference? *J Hum Lactat* 28(3):380–8.

Gatrell CJ (2007) Secrets and lies: breastfeeding and professional paid work. *Soc Sci Med* 65(2):393–404.

Gonidakis F, Rabavilas AD, Varsou E, Kreatsas G, Christodoulou GN (2008) A 6-month study of postpartum depression and related factors in Athens Greece. *Compr Psychiatry* Jun 30;49(3):275–82.

Grassley J, Eschiti V (2008) Grandmother breastfeeding support: what do mothers need and want? *Birth* 35(4):329–35.

Guardian (2018) Breastfeeding support services failing mothers due to cuts (27/07/18). www.theguardian.com/lifeandstyle/2018/jul/27/breastfeeding-support-services-failing-mothers-due-to-cuts

Harries V, Brown A (2019a) The association between baby care books that promote strict care routines and infant feeding, night-time care, and maternal–infant interactions. Matern Child Nutr e12858.

Harries V, Brown A (2019b) The association between use of infant parenting books that promote strict routines, and maternal depression, self-efficacy, and parenting confidence. *Early Child Dev Care* 189(8):1339–50.

Hauck YL, Fenwick J, Dhaliwal SS (2011) The association between women's perceptions of professional support and problems experienced on breastfeeding cessation: a Western Australian study. *J Hum Lactat* 27(1):49–57.

Henderson JJ, Evans SF, Straton JA, Priest SR, Hagan R (2003) Impact of postnatal depression on breastfeeding duration. *Birth* 30(3):175–80.

Henderson L, McMillan B, Green JM, Renfrew MJ (2011) Men and infant feeding: perceptions of embarrassment, sexuality, and social conduct in white low-income British men. Birth 38(1):61–70.

Hoddinott P, Pill R (1999) Qualitative study of decisions about infant feeding among women in east end of London. *BMJ* 318(7175):30–4.

Hoddinott P, Craig LC, Britten J, McInnes RM (2012) A serial qualitative interview study of infant feeding experiences: idealism meets realism. *BMJ Open* 2(2): e000504.

Kendall-Tackett K (2007) A new paradigm for depression in new mothers: the central role of inflammation and how breastfeeding and anti-inflammatory treatments protect maternal mental health. *Int Breastfeed J* 2(1):6.

Konner M (1977) Infancy among the Kalahari Desert San. *Culture and Infancy: Variations in the Human Experience.* New York: Academic Press, pp. 287–328.

Kosmala-Anderson J, Wallace LM (2006) Breastfeeding works: the role of employers in supporting women who wish to breastfeed and work in four organisations in England. *J Public Health* 28(3):183–91.

Lawrence RM, Lawrence RA (2001) Given the benefits of breastfeeding, what contraindications exist? *Pediatr Clin* 48(1):235–51.

Leigh B, Milgrom J (2008) Risk factors for antenatal depression, postnatal depression and parenting stress. *BMC Psychiatry* 8(1):24.

Maternity Action UK (2018) Continuing to breastfeed when you return to work. https://maternityaction.org.uk

McAndrew F, Thompson J, Fellows L (2012) *Infant Feeding Survey 2010.* Leeds: Health and Social Care Information Centre.

McKenna JJ, Ball HL, Gettler LT (2007) Mother–infant cosleeping, breastfeeding and sudden infant death syndrome: what biological anthropology has discovered about normal infant sleep and pediatric sleep medicine. *Am J Phys Anthropol* 134(S45):133–61.

McClellan HL, Hepworth AR, Garbin CP, Rowan MK, Deacon J, Hartmann PE, Geddes DT (2012) Nipple pain during breastfeeding with or without visible trauma. *J Hum Lactat* 28(4):511–521.

Neville MC, Morton J, Umemura S (2001) Lactogenesis: the transition from pregnancy to lactation. *Pediatr Clin* 48(1):35–52.

Paris R, Dubus N (2005) Staying connected while nurturing an infant: a challenge of new motherhood. *Fam Relat* 54(1):72–83.

Park CW, Milberg S, Lawson R (1991) Evaluation of brand extensions: the role of product feature similarity and brand concept consistency. *J Consumer Res* 18(2):185–93.

Pontes CM, Osório MM, Alexandrino AC (2009) Building a place for the father as an ally for breast feeding. *Midwifery* 25(2):195–202.

Renfrew MJ, Pokhrel S, Quigley M (2012) *Preventing Disease and Saving Resources: The Potential Contribution of Increasing Breastfeeding Rates in the UK.* UNICEF.

Rollins NC, Bhandari N, Hajeebhoy N (2016) Why invest, and what will it take to improve breastfeeding practices? *Lancet* 387(10017):491–504.

Rosenberg KD, Eastham CA, Kasehagen LJ, Sandoval AP (2008) Marketing infant formula through hospitals: the impact of commercial hospital discharge packs on breastfeeding. *Am J Public Health* 98(2):290–5.

Sherriff N, Hall V (2011) Engaging and supporting fathers to promote breastfeeding: a new role for health visitors? *Scand J Caring Sci* 25(3):467–75.

Shildrick M (1997) *Leaky Bodies and Boundaries: Feminism, Postmodernism and (Bio) Ethics.* London: Routledge.

Susin LR, Giugliani ER, Kummer SC (2005) Influence of grandmothers on breastfeeding practices. *Rev Saude Publica* 39(2):141–7.

Swanson V, Power KG (2005) Initiation and continuation of breastfeeding: theory of planned behaviour. *J Adv Nurs* 50(3):272–82.

Thomson G, Dykes F (2011) Women's sense of coherence related to their infant feeding experiences. *Matern Child Nutr* 7(2):160–74.

Thomson G, Crossland N, Dykes F (2012) Giving me hope: women's reflections on a breastfeeding peer support service. *Matern Child Nutr* 8(3):340–53.

Trevathan W, Trevathan W (2010) *Ancient Bodies, Modern Lives: How Evolution has Shaped Women's Health.* Oxford University Press.

Trickey H, Totelin L, Sanders J (2017) Nain, mam and me: historical artefacts as prompts for reminiscence, reflection and conversation about feeding babies. A qualitative development study. *Res All* 1(1):64–83.

Victora CG, Bahl R, Barros AJ (2016) Breastfeeding in the 21st century: epidemiology, mechanisms, and lifelong effect. *Lancet* 387(10017):475–90.

Walker K (2017) What issues to lesbian co-mothers face in their transition to parenthood? *NCT Perspectives* 34. www.nct.org.uk/sites/default/files/related_documents/Walker%20 K%20What%20issues%20do%20lesbian%20co-mothers%20face%20in%20their%20 transition%20to%20parenthood.pdf

WHO (1981) *International Code of Marketing of Breast-Milk Substitutes.* Geneva: WHO. www.who.int/nutrition/publications/code_english.pdf

4   Contraindications to breastfeeding

Wendy Jones

There are few absolute contraindications to breastfeeding other than the wishes of the mother. However, we need to be aware of the limited medical conditions and medications which impact on the decision so that families are empowered to make evidence-based decisions.

Some mothers choose not to breastfeed and that decision should be supported. However, there are also a group of women who will be advised not to breastfeed because of a medical condition or medication. These situations are rare but the impact for a family may be considerable if they had decided antenatally to breastfeed the baby. The parents should be provided with a full explanation as to why breastfeeding is not recommended so that they do not simply feel disempowered.

A campaign has been launched recently by the Hospital Feeding Network, GP Infant Feeding Network and Breastfeeding Network with the support of UK Drugs in Lactation Advisory Service (UKDILAS) with the title #dontsaystoplookit up to encourage professionals not to rely solely on the *British National Formulary* (BNF) in line with the prescribing recommendation in National Institute for Health and Care Excellence PH11 guidance (NICE 2014) and to use expert sources.

Medical contraindications to breastfeeding

Every baby is given a newborn blood spot screening (heel prick test) at 5 days of age to identify if the baby has one of nine conditions. Some of the conditions tested for have implications for breastfeeding; the most common are described below.

Phenylketonuria (PKU)

PKU is an inherited condition affecting one in every 10,000 live births each year (Hardelid et al. 2008). It is due to a deficiency of the enzyme phenylalanine hydroxylase responsible for the metabolism of phenylalanine into tyrosine. Unchecked, the levels of phenylalanine accumulate and interfere with brain development, resulting in mental and growth retardation. Breastfeeding can continue whilst blood levels are monitored (Kanufre et al. 2007). Levels of phenylalanine in human milk were found to be lower than in any formula on the market (Banta-Wright et al. 2014). Babies with PKU who are breastfed along with formula milk containing low phenylalanine were found to have a lower phenylalanine intake and higher IQ score than infants fed only on formula containing low phenylalanine (Riordan and Auerbach 2004). A literature review covering large numbers of mothers who breastfed an infant with PKU suggested that the vast majority of women in this situation manage to continue to breastfeed their infant successfully, and without problems in the infant (Banta-Wright et al. 2014)

Galactosaemia

Galactosaemia occurs in about 1 in 45,000 births (Walter et al. 1999). It is a deficiency of enzyme galactose-1-phosphate uridyl transferase transmitted as an autosomal-recessive trait. The liver enzyme that converts galactose to glucose is absent, so the baby is unable to metabolise lactose. The infants appear normal at birth but often have feeding difficulties, with jaundice, enlarged liver, lethargy, irritability, vomiting and poor weight gain (Walker 2006). Without treatment mental retardation develops. Galactosaemia is one of the few instances where breastfeeding needs to stop immediately to be replaced by galactose-free formula milk. Approximately one in every 19,000 infants born in Ireland may have this condition. However, it is particularly common among infants born to Traveller parents, in whom the incidence is approximately 1 in 450 births. Babies of the Traveller community are offered the Beutler test on day 1 of life and are fed galactose-free feed (soya-based) formula and not breastfed until the result of the test is available. This protects the infant if he/she has the condition (UCD School of Public Health and Population 2010).

Maple syrup urine disease

Maple syrup urine disease is a life-threatening condition if not detected and treated early. It is an autosomal-recessive disorder caused by a defect in the metabolism of the three branched-chain amino acids. It affects approximately one live birth in every 185,000 per year worldwide (Walker 2006). A delay in diagnosis longer than 14 days is invariably associated with mental retardation and cerebral palsy. Treatment relies on dietary restriction of branched-chain amino acids for life. In a study one baby was breastfed under controlled conditions after the control of acute metabolic problems. The baby continued with breastfeeding on demand and with the addition of a special essential amino acid mixture. However, the baby experienced difficulties both in metabolic control and in insufficiency of breast milk, resulting in termination of breastfeeding (Huner et al. 2005).

The other conditions identified by the heel prick test are:

- sickle cell disease (incidence 1 in 2,000): breastfeeding can continue;
- cystic fibrosis (incidence 1 in 2,500): may need additional nutrient-dense feeds;
- congenital hypothyroidism (incidence 1 in 3,000): breastfeeding can continue;
- medium-chain acyl-coenzyme A dehydrogenase deficiency (MCADD): (incidence 1 in 100,000–150,000): may need additional sweet drinks during illness;
- isovaleric acidaemia (IVA) (incidence 1 in 100,000–150,000): breastfeeding can continue;
- glutaric aciduria type 1 (GA1) (incidence 1 in 100,000–150,000): breastfeeding can continue;
- homocystinuria (pyridoxine-unresponsive) (HCU) (incidence 1 in 100,000–150,000): breastfeeding can continue.

In all conditions the baby may need to be monitored.

Medical conditions where breastfeeding may be contraindicated but not identified by the blood spot test

Hepatitis C

Hepatitis C is a liver infection caused by the hepatitis C virus (HCV), transmitted by blood from an infected person. There is no documented evidence that breastfeeding spreads HCV. In one study of 17 HCV-positive mothers, 11 of the 17 had hepatitis C antibodies present in milk, but none had RNA particles of hepatitis C, indicating that the virus itself was not present in milk (Grayson et al. 1995). Therefore, having hepatitis C infection is not a contraindication to breastfeed. However, if the mother develops cracked or bleeding nipples there is in theory a risk of transmission so she may be advised to stop breastfeeding until the cracks have resolved through the use of moist wound healing (Mast 2004). She will need to express to maintain her supply and should be referred for local, expert face-to-face support to resolve the poor latch which resulted in the damage.

Hepatitis B

This virus is transmitted through contact with infected blood and bodily fluids. Hepatitis B antigen has been detected in breastmilk. However, women infected with hepatitis B can breastfeed and this does not confer any additional risk for the transmission of hepatitis B to the baby over and above birth. Infants of infected mothers should receive a course of hepatitis B vaccine soon after birth. Babies are usually given the second dose of the vaccine 1–2 months after the first dose, and the third dose by the time they are 18 months old (Hale and Rowe 2017).

Human immunodeficiency virus (HIV)

In the UK and other high-income settings, the safest way to feed infants born to women with HIV is with formula milk, as there is no ongoing risk of HIV exposure after birth. The British HIV Association (2018) therefore continues to recommend that women living with HIV feed their babies with formula milk. In 2010 WHO guidelines on HIV and infant feeding for the first time recommended the use of anti-retroviral drugs to prevent postnatal transmission of HIV through breastfeeding. This resulted in a major change from an individualised counselling approach toward a public health approach regarding how maternal and child health services should routinely promote and support infant feeding practices among mothers living with HIV (WHO 2016).

UK guidance has been reviewed in the light of data showing the protective effect of antiretroviral therapy during breastfeeding.

> BHIVA/CHIVA [Children's HIV Association] acknowledge that, in the UK, the risk of mother-to-child transmission through exclusive breastfeeding from a woman who is on HAART [highly active antiretroviral therapy] and has a consistently undetectable HIV viral load is likely to be low but emphasise that this risk has not yet been quantified. Therefore, avoidance of breastfeeding is still the best and safest option in the UK to prevent mother-to-child transmission of HIV.
>
> (British HIV Association 2018)

Herpes simplex virus (HSV)

In infants HSV can be severe, resulting in high rates of mortality and morbidity. Mothers with herpes can continue to breastfeed as long as there are no lesions present on the breasts and if lesions elsewhere on the body are carefully covered. Every precaution needs to be taken to prevent infants from being exposed to the herpes virus and appropriate hand hygiene should be stressed.

Medication contraindicated during breastfeeding

There are few situations where there is not a suitable drug to use to treat a breastfeeding mother and allow her to continue feeding as normal (Jones 2018).

Drugs which are absolutely contraindicated during breastfeeding

- antineoplastics (although in theory it is possible to re-establish lactation after treatment);
- lithium (except with very close monitoring of the baby);
- oral retinoids;
- iodine;
- amiodarone;
- methotrexate (other than for management of ectopic pregnancy);
- gold salts.

Drugs which should be prescribed with caution

- combined oral contraceptive before 3 months (reduces milk supply in some mothers);
- loop diuretics – may reduce supply;
- centrally acting drugs – may cause the baby to be drowsy;
- medication containing codeine;
- drugs on which there are no pharmacokinetic data and new drugs with which there is limited experience;
- sustained-release preparations or long-half-life drugs in neonates as this may lead to accumulation (e.g. fluconazole, pethidine).

Drugs which may be purchased by the mother which should be used with caution

- pseudoephedrine in cold remedies (reduction in milk supply);
- herbal products (e.g. cannabidiol (CBD) oil) on which there are usually limited data.

When is a drug contraindicated in breastfeeding prescribed?

If it is essential to prescribe for a mother a medication which is contraindicated in breastfeeding, it is recommended that the mother seek support from a qualified breastfeeding expert who can help her to wean the baby on to an alternative milk and reduce her own supply. Ideally, weaning from the breast should take place slowly to avoid the discomfort as well as risk of blocked ducts and mastitis. However, occasionally it will be necessary to wean abruptly. Weaning against her original wishes may be upsetting for a mother and her distress should not be dismissed but supported with empathy. Whether she has breastfed for 6 days, 6 weeks or 6 years breastfeeding has been chosen by the mother and this should not be undervalued so that she can look back on the decision positively. Sometimes it may be possible to provide the family with donor breastmilk, e.g. following diagnosis of cancer antenatally via the Human Milk Foundation, and the contact can be offered.

References

Banta-Wright SA, Press N, Knafl KA, Steiner RD, Houck GM (2014) Breastfeeding infants with phenylketonuria in the United States and Canada. *Breastfeed Med* 9(3):142–8.

British HIV Association (2018) BHIVA guidelines on the management of HIV in pregnancy and postpartum. www.bhiva.org/pregnancy-guidelines

Grayson ML, Braniff KM, Bowden DS, Turnidge JD (1995) Breastfeeding and the risk of vertical transmission of hepatitis C virus. *Med J Aust* 163(2):107.

Hale TW, Rowe HE (2017) *Medications and Mothers' Milk 2017.* Springer.

Hardelid P, Cortina-Borja M, Munro A, Jones H, Cleary M, Champion MP, Foo Y, Scriver CR, Dezateux C (2008) The birth prevalence of PKU in populations of European, South Asian and sub-Saharan African ancestry living in South East England. *Ann Hum Genet* 72:65–71.

Huner G, Baykal T, Demir F, Demirkol M (2005) Breastfeeding experience in inborn errors of metabolism other than phenylketonuria. *J Inherit Metab Dis* 28(4):457–65.

Jones W (2018) *Breastfeeding and Medication.* Routledge.

Kanufre VC, Starling AL, Leão E, Aguiar MJ, Santos JS, Soares RD, Silveira AM (2007) Breastfeeding in the treatment of children with phenylketonuria. *J Pediatr (Rio J)* 83(5):447–52.

Mast EE (2004) Mother-to-infant hepatitis C virus transmission and breastfeeding. *Adv Exp Med Biol* 554:211–16.

McAndrew F, Thompson J, Fellows L, Large A, Speed M. Renfrew MJ (2012) *Infant Feeding Survey.* NHS Information Service.

NICE (2014) *Maternal and Child Nutrition.* PH11. London: NICE.

Riordan JM, Auerbach KG (2004) *Breastfeeding and Human Lactation,* 4th ed. Sudbury: Jones and Bartlett.

UCD School of Public Health and Population (2010) 'Breastfeeding is natural, but it's not the norm in Ireland'. An assessment of the barriers to breastfeeding and the service needs of families and communities in Ireland with low breastfeeding rates. www.hse.ie/eng/about/who/healthwellbeing/our-priority-programmes/child-health-and-wellbeing/breastfeeding-healthy-childhood-programme/research-and-reports-breastfeeding/barriers-to-breasfteeding-ucd-report-2010.pdf

Walker M (2006) *Breastfeeding Management for the Clinician.* Jones & Bartlett.

Walter JH, Collins JE, Leonard JV (1999) Recommendations for the management of galactosaemia. *Arch Dis Child* 80:93–6.

WHO (2016) Updates on HIV and infant feeding. The duration of breastfeeding and support from health services to improve feeding practices among mothers living with HIV. https://www.who.int/maternal_child_adolescent/documents/hiv-infant-feeding-2016/en/

5 Breastfeeding and infant sleep – what medical practitioners need to know

Helen L. Ball

- Infant sleep is hugely variable in terms of 24-hour duration, and changes over time.
- For many decades the model for infant sleep science was based on formula-fed infants, sleeping alone, in a prone position.
- Human infants are unusually helpless at birth, requiring prolonged care characterised by close mother–infant contact 24 hours per day with frequent suckling. This benefits both baby and mother.
- Despite popular perceptions, feed-type does not affect total sleep time, but does affect sleep fragmentation (breastfed infants wake more frequently to feed at night).
- Mothers of breastfed infants manage the sleep disruption of night-time feeding by sleeping with their babies, and bed-share in a very characteristic manner.
- Separation of breastfeeding mother–infant dyads at night interferes with breastfeeding initiation and duration.
- Breastfed infants exhibit a very low rate of sudden infant death syndrome (SIDS) which is not dramatically increased by bed-sharing so long as hazardous practices are avoided.
- There is a wide range of resources available to help practitioners discuss sleep and breastfeeding issues with parents before and after their baby is born.

Does breastfeeding affect sleep, and does sleep affect breastfeeding? The answers to both these questions are largely, 'Yes'; however much of the relevant research is recent, and evidence-based information on the relationship between breastfeeding and sleep has not been part of the training of many clinicians or health professionals. This chapter summarises the key issues medical professionals should be aware of when responding to queries or giving advice on these topics.

Studies of infant sleep began in earnest in the 1950s: infant sleep characteristics were 'defined' based on studies of formula-fed babies sleeping alone, and sleep was 'measured' via maternal reports of whether she was aware that the baby woke in the night (Moore and Ucko 1957). Research at this time focused upon ascertaining 'normative values' for infant sleep to produce charts depicting sleep benchmarks (Kleitman and Engelmann 1953; Parmelee et al. 1964). These 'normative values' have changed dramatically over the decades with more objective measures: we now know infants exhibit a wide range of sleep needs throughout their first year (Galland et al. 2012), and that sleep consolidation follows different trajectories for different infants (Henderson et al. 2010).

Sleep scientists did not consider the role of infant feeding in their studies until relatively recently (indeed, not until women began working in this field, e.g. Elias et al. 1986), while studies of the sleep of parents caring for infants do not appear in the literature until the end of the last century (e.g. Keefe 1988; Horiuchi and Nishihara 1999), with the majority being published during the last decade. Before considering this research, however, it is important to think about the biological constraints on human babies and their mothers that shape the outcomes for breastfeeding and sleep.

The evolved characteristics of human infants and maternal care

As mammals, the defining characteristic of our taxonomic class is producing milk for our babies, but as a species humans also have other unique defining characteristics: bipedalism and unusually large brains (Trevathan and Rosenberg 2016). Understanding how human babies sleep involves appreciating how these features have shaped infancy and infant care, so we begin by considering the implications of the uniquely human, and shared mammalian, characteristics of human babies.

There are three broad mammalian groups, all of which produce milk for their infants: monotremes (e.g. echidna and platypus); marsupials (e.g. koalas, kangaroos and possums); and placental (or eutherian) mammals, which includes all those mammals whose infants are sustained in early life in a uterus with a placenta rather than in an egg (monotremes) or a pouch (marsupials). Biologists divide the placental mammals into two types (altricial and precocial) based on the developmental state of the infant at birth. Altricial infants experience a short gestation period, and are born into litters of multiple siblings, with undeveloped sensory organs (they can't see, hear or call), and are usually hairless and weak. In contrast, precocial infants are born singly or in pairs after a much longer gestation period and are therefore born in a more well-developed state, being able to see, hear, call, thermoregulate (being covered with hair/fur) and to stand independently or actively cling to their mothers shortly after birth.

The state of these infants at birth affects the ways they are cared for: mothers of altricial infants (e.g. mice, rabbits, cats and dogs) cache their newborns in nests which provide safety and warmth, and leave them hidden while they forage, often for many hours a day. They produce milk that has high fat content and satiates their babies for long periods. In some species mothers only return to the nest once or twice per day to feed their babies, which spend several weeks sleeping and growing. By the time they emerge from the nest altricial infants have increased their birthweight many times and have fully functioning sensory and locomotor capabilities. In contrast, mothers of precocial infants (e.g. elephants, horses, primates), use a 'carry or follow strategy': infants remain with the mother while she forages, and she provides them with safety and warmth. Females produce milk that is low in fat, but high in sugar, providing their babies with energy. Because precocial infants are in constant proximity to their mother they do not need to be able to sustain long periods between feeds (Lozoff and Brittenham 1979).

Human babies are born singly or in pairs following a prolonged gestation and are born with well-developed sensory organs, being able to see, hear and call. Human mothers produce milk that provides energy (sugar) rather than fat. By these criteria human infants are precocial along with all other primates; however human infants are incapable of standing, walking or even clinging to their mother for several months following birth. Humans therefore produce unusually helpless precocial babies – a situation that arose as a consequence of our evolutionary history (Trevathan and Rosenberg 2016). The two defining characteristics of humans – bipedalism (walking on two legs) and encephalisation (massively large brains) – have resulted in human babies being born before their brains are sufficiently developed for competent neuromuscular control. It is debated whether the key constraint on human prenatal development was the size of the baby's head versus the bipedal pelvic outlet or was the ability of female metabolism to sustain the energetic demands of a fetus with a larger brain. Whichever way it happened, human babies are born with more immature brains relative to their adult brain size (25%) than are all other primates (50%) (Trevathan and Rosenberg 2016). During their first year of life the brains of human infants grow more rapidly than any other primate, only slowing down after 12 months of age (Martin 2007).

Aspects of infant biology linked to sleep, therefore, involve the need for close proximity to the mother and frequent feeding day and night, plus rapid brain growth necessitating a high proportion of rapid eye movement (REM) sleep (when neural connections are made) (McKenna et al. 2007). The biology of early infancy therefore predicts that human babies should wake to feed periodically during the night, that this might persist throughout the first year of life due to the energetic needs of rapid brain growth, and that they will spend a large proportion of sleep time in REM sleep and less time in quiet sleep than they will as they mature. Additionally, babies are born with no circadian clock, and it takes several months for a day–night rhythm to become established (Joseph et al. 2015).

The above biological view of infant sleep is very different from the cultural expectations of infant sleep in most Western societies. For the past century views of infant sleep have been shaped by cultural and political perspectives emphasising early independence, self-control and self-reliance. That crying is 'good for babies', that they will be 'spoiled' if picked up or become 'clingy' if allowed access to their parents at night are all cultural constructs reflecting historical ideologies of the past century, with no evidence from developmental biology (Hardyment 1983; Ball et al. 2019).

The sleep of breastfed babies and breastfeeding mums

Parental interviews and focus groups about the relationship between infant feeding and sleeping reveal contradictory views: on the one hand many parents express firm beliefs that giving babies formula helps to reduce night waking (Ball 2003) while others consider this an 'old-fashioned notion' (Rudzik and Ball 2016). Studies based on parental reports of infant night-waking perpetuate the view that feeding infants formula is associated with more sleep, deeper sleep and earlier sleep consolidation (Moore and Ucko 1957); however objective studies using actigraphy find no differences in the amount of sleep obtained per night by infants based on feed-type (Tikotsky et al. 2009; Rudzik et al. 2018). Quillin and Glenn (2004), Doan et al. (2007) and Montgomery-Downs et al. (2010) likewise confirm that breastfeeding and formula-feeding mothers obtain the same amounts of sleep per night. However, Rudzik et al. (2018) found that perceptions of sleep by the two groups differed widely, with mothers of formula-fed babies reporting their infants experienced much longer night-time sleep bouts than did mothers of breastfed babies. This phenomenon may be related to sleep proximity, the effects of breastfeeding hormones or to expectations.

Although breastfeeders get the same or more total sleep per night, feeding-related sleep fragmentation means an experience of poorer sleep quality for breastfeeding mothers in some cases (Ball 2003; McBean and Montgomery-Downs 2014). As a consequence, the vast majority of breastfeeding mothers tend to sleep with their babies in their bed as a strategy to cope with sleep disruption for at least some of the time (Ball 2003; Ateah and Hamelin 2008; Rudzik and Ball 2016). Numerous studies have confirmed that, although bed-sharing breastfeeding mothers wake frequently to feed, they also wake for shorter periods and fall back to sleep more rapidly (Mosko et al. 1997b) when compared to not bed-sharing. It is unsurprising that breastfeeding mothers comprise the largest group of co-sleepers. Of 34 studies exploring maternal reasons for co-sleeping, 26 reported breastfeeding as the key reason (Salm-Ward 2015). It is important to understand, therefore, that bed-sharing is a common night-time care strategy for breastfeeding mothers and babies which supports their evolved biology (Ball and Russell 2012; McKenna and Gettler 2016; Ball 2017).

When parents in Western countries are interviewed about sleeping with their baby they express various reasons for doing so, such as deeply rooted cultural or religious beliefs and parenting philosophies, physiological links between lactation and night-time breastfeeding and a biological compulsion that drives the urge for close contact (Ball 2002; Ateah and Hamelin 2008; Culver 2009; Salm-Ward 2015; Crane and Ball 2016). On a practical level they explain that sleeping with the baby makes night-time care easier, helps them to monitor the baby, providing comfort, and yet obtaining sleep (Ball 2002; Ball 2003; Rudzik and Ball 2016). Sometimes parents report having nowhere else to put their baby at night, or that they have fallen asleep with their baby unintentionally (Ball 2002; Ateah and Hamelin 2008; Volpe et al. 2013). Despite decades of advice to avoid mother–baby sleep contact (for various reasons), 20–25% of US and UK babies under 3 months of age share a bed with a parent for sleep on any given night (Blair and Ball 2004; McCoy et al. 2004) and during their first 3 months 40–70% of babies in those Western societies surveyed to date have done so (Gibson et al. 2000; Rigda et al. 2000; Willinger et al. 2003; Blair and Ball 2004; Ateah and Hamelin 2008; Hauck et al. 2008; Santos et al. 2009). Recent studies have found that mother–infant bed-sharing in low-risk circumstances is no more hazardous for babies than sleeping in a cot (Blair et al. 2014), and that advising parents against bed-sharing does not reduce its prevalence (Moon et al. 2017).

Do sleeping arrangements affect breastfeeding?

It may be surprising to learn that small variations in sleep location have substantial consequences for the functioning of maternal lactation biology. In a randomised video trial carried out on the postnatal ward of a large northern hospital in England we randomly allocated mothers and babies to: (1) normal rooming-in with a standard bassinet; (2) bed-sharing with a side-car crib attached to the mother's bed; and (3) bed-sharing directly in the mother's bed with a mesh cot-side to protect against falls. We found that infant sleep location affects infant feed frequency among breastfeeding mother–infant dyads in the immediate postpartum with in-bed and side-car crib dyads feeding twice as frequently throughout the night as those receiving the normal bassinet (Ball et al. 2006; Ball and Klingaman 2007; Ball 2008).

This is important due to the effect of feed frequency in modulating human lactation physiology, with earlier and more vigorous onset of lactogenesis II (LII, copious milk production) (Salariya et al. 1978; Tennekoon et al. 1994; Riordan 2011). LII is triggered when prolactin levels in maternal plasma reach a threshold accumulated over several days (Neville 2001). As a prolactin surge is experienced with every feed or attempted feed, and as each surge in prolactin declines after 45 minutes, repeated frequent feeding day and night results in circulating blood prolactin rising swiftly, and earlier attainment of the threshold that triggers onset of LII (Neville 2001; Neville and Morton 2001). Contemporary postnatal hospital environments that enforce mother–infant separation at night (even separation via the wall of a hospital bassinet) therefore exert physiological and psychological influences on the behavioural and biological relationship between mother and baby (Ball 2008). These findings support McKenna and Gettler's (2016) proposal that breastfeeding and co-sleeping form an adaptive and mutually reinforcing behavioural complex that they have termed 'breastsleeping'.

Sleep contact facilitates night-time breastfeeding and is associated with more frequent night-time feeds (which promote milk production) and more months of breastfeeding (Santos et al. 2009; Huang et al. 2013; Ball et al. 2016). Although some authors have viewed this relationship as evidence that bed-sharing protects against early weaning, the association does not reveal the direction of causality. In a study of 870 mothers, we found that those who commenced bed-sharing within the first 3 months were twice as likely still to be breastfeeding 6 months post-birth than if they did not (Figure 5.1); but also that mothers who chose to bed-share were those with the strongest prenatal intent to breastfeed to 6 months or beyond (Howel and Ball 2013; Ball et al. 2016). These data support the view that bed-sharing is a strategy used

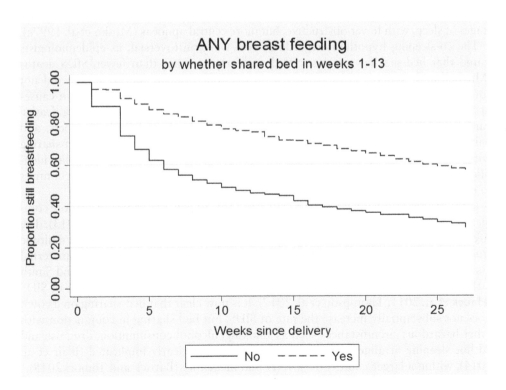

Figure 5.1 Bed-sharing is strongly associated with breastfeeding continuation
Source: Ball (2016).

by breastfeeding mothers to reduce the costs (such as sleep disruption) of prolonged breastfeeding (Tully and Ball 2013). Prevention of bed-sharing is likely, therefore, to undermine breastfeeding goals (Ball 2003; Blair et al. 2010; Bartick and Smith 2014).

Sudden infant death syndrome (SIDS) and safer sleep guidance

The relationship between night-time breastfeeding, frequent feeding and bed-sharing of course raises concerns about infant sleep safety and SIDS. Although the cause of SIDS remains unknown, epidemiological studies have identified a strong association with infant sleep position, leading to campaigns that informed parents to sleep babies on their backs (Gilbert et al. 2005). Further infant care practices prevalent in Western countries (where SIDS rates were high) were subsequently scrutinised, such as use of pacifiers, soft bedding and head covering. In the late 1980s anthropologists noted how poorly Western sleep arrangements met the human infant's unique biological and behavioural needs (McKenna 1986; Konner and Super 1987), with babies predominantly sleeping alone in cribs in separate rooms from their parents. In suggesting that one explanation for SIDS could be the unusual Western practice of separating babies and mothers at night, McKenna proposed that infants experiencing close sleep contact may be protected from apnoeic pauses and blunted arousal by maternal sounds, movements and breathing (McKenna 1986; McKenna et al. 1993). Infants experience dramatic changes in their breathing control around 3 months of age which make them particularly vulnerable to unpredictable breathing cessation (Mosko et al. 1997a); in a polysomnographic study of breastfeeding mothers and babies McKenna and colleagues demonstrated that sleep contact promoted regular night-time interaction and lighter stages of sleep, with fewer obstructive, but more central apnoeas (Mosko et al. 1997a).

The co-sleeping hypothesis regarding SIDS was controversial, as epidemiologists found that bed-sharing was associated with more, rather than fewer, SIDS deaths (Mitchell and Scragg 1993). However, these initial epidemiological studies did not consider the interaction between bed-sharing and smoking and other known causes of SIDS, or the protective effects of breastfeeding; definitions of 'bed-sharing deaths' varied widely, encompassing sofa-sharing, sleep-sharing with siblings or pets, and babies returned to a crib (Cote 2006). Although it became clear that room-sharing with parents was protective (Scragg et al. 1996), several epidemiological studies identified bed-sharing as a dangerous activity, prompting strict guidance in many countries to dissuade parents from bed-sharing (Bartick and Smith 2014).

In time the relationship between bed-sharing and SIDS was revealed to be more complex than initially assumed (Fetherston and Leach 2012; Ball and Volpe 2013). The strong relationship between bed-sharing and breastfeeding was replicated in multiple studies, suggesting that a 'Never bed-share' message may not only hinder maternal and child health promotion by impeding breastfeeding (Ball 2003; Bartick and Smith 2014), but also impede SIDS reduction itself, as breastfeeding halves the risk of SIDS (Hauck et al. 2011; Thompson et al. 2017). It is now clear that bed-sharing on its own does not substantially increase the rate of SIDS, but bed-sharing in conjunction with other hazardous circumstances such as smoking, alcohol consumption, drug use and ad hoc sleeping arrangements such as sofa-sharing is clearly implicated (Blair et al. 2014), within a larger context of poverty and inequality (Bartick and Tomori 2018).

Breastfeeding babies who sleep with their mothers in the absence of known hazards have no greater SIDS risk than if they sleep in a cot. Mothers protect them from

Table 5.1 Resources to support discussion of sleep for breastfeeding mothers and babies

Resource	Website
Baby Sleep Information Source (Basis)	www.BasisOnline.org.uk
UNICEF Caring for your baby at night plus health professional's guide	www.unicef.org.uk/babyfriendly/baby-friendly-resources/sleep-and-night-time-resources/caring-for-your-baby-at-night/
NICE guidance on co-sleeping and SIDS	www.nice.org.uk/guidance/cg37/evidence/full-guideline-addendum-485782238
Infant sleep safety materials	www.lullabytrust.org.uk/professionals/publications/
Co-sleeping and SIDS: a guide for health professionals	www.unicef.org.uk/babyfriendly/baby-friendly-resources/sleep-and-night-time-resources/co-sleeping-and-sids/
Where might my baby sleep?	www.basisonline.org.uk/where-might-my-baby-sleep/

potential physiological stressors such as airway covering and overheating by their characteristic sleep position (curled around their babies, making a constrained sleep space with their bodies) documented in multiple video studies, and their continued vigilance via micro-arousals which prompt regular infant arousals throughout the night (Mosko 1997a, 1997b; Ball 2006; Baddock et al. 2019). Further research is needed to determine whether these protective and apparently inherent behaviours can be taught to non-breastfeeders.

Overall the research conducted to date on sleep and breastfeeding indicates that close night-time proximity facilitates breastfeeding initiation and supports women to continue breastfeeding. Breastfeeding is not associated with less sleep for mother and baby but does affect sleep fragmentation. Breastfeeding mothers choose to bed-share in order to facilitate night-time feeding (breastsleeping) and it is increasingly recommended that ways to facilitate safe bed-sharing should be incorporated into guidelines for postnatal care (e.g. Fetherston and Leach 2012; Drever-Smith et al. 2013; Crenshaw 2014; Feldman-Winter and Goldsmith 2016) (Table 5.1).

References

Ateah CA, Hamelin KJ (2008) Maternal bedsharing practices, experiences, and awareness of risks. *J Obstet Gynecol Neonatal Nurs* 37(3):274–81.

Baddock SA, Purnell MT, Blair PS, Pease AS, Elder DE, Galland BC (2019) The influence of bed-sharing on infant physiology, breastfeeding and behaviour: a systematic review. *Sleep Med Rev* 43:106–17.

Ball HL (2002) Reasons to bed-share: why parents sleep with their infants. *J Reprod Infant Psychol* 20(4):207–21.

Ball HL (2003) Breastfeeding, bed-sharing, and infant sleep. *Birth* 30(3):181–8.

Ball HL (2006) Parent–infant bed-sharing behavior: effects of feeding type and presence of father. *Hum Nature* 17(3):301–18.

Ball HL (2008) Evolutionary paediatrics: a case study in applying Darwinian medicine. In: Elton S, O'Higgins P (eds) *Medicine and Evolution: Current Applications, Future Prospects.* London: Taylor and Francis, pp. 125–50.

Ball HL (2017) Evolution-informed maternal–infant health. *Nature Ecol Evol* 1(3):0073.

Ball HL, Klingaman K (2007) Breastfeeding and mother–infant sleep proximity: implications for infant care. In: Trevathan WR, Smith EO, McKenna J (eds) *Evolutionary Medicine and Health*. New York: Oxford University Press, pp. 152–72.

Ball HL, Russell CK (2012) Night-time nurturing: an evolutionary perspective on breastfeeding and sleep. In: Narváez D, Panksepp J, Schore A, Gleason T (eds) *Evolution, Early Experience and Human Development: From Research to Practice and Policy*. Oxford: Oxford University Press, pp. 241–61.

Ball HL, Volpe LE (2013) Sudden infant death syndrome (SIDS) risk reduction and infant sleep location – moving the discussion forward. *Soc Sci Med* 79:84–91.

Ball HL, Ward-Platt MP, Heslop E, Leech SJ, Brown KA (2006) Randomised trial of infant sleep location on the postnatal ward. *Arch Dis Child* 91(12):1005–10.

Ball HL, Howel D, Bryant A, Best E, Russell C, Ward-Platt M (2016) Bed-sharing by breastfeeding mothers: who bed-shares and what is the relationship with breastfeeding duration? *Acta Paediatr* 105(6):628–34.

Ball HL, Tomori C, McKenna JJ (2019) Towards an integrated anthropology of infant sleep. *Am Anthropologist* 121(3):595–612.

Bartick M, Smith LJ (2014) Speaking out on safe sleep: evidence-based infant sleep recommendations. *Breastfeed Med* 9(9):417–22.

Bartick M, Tomori C (2018) Sudden infant death and social justice: a syndemics approach. *Matern Child Nutr* e12652.

Bartick M, Tomori C, Ball HL (2018) Babies in boxes and the missing links on safe sleep: human evolution and cultural revolution. *Matern Child Nutr* 14(2):e12544.

Blair PS, Ball HL (2004) The prevalence and characteristics associated with parent–infant bed-sharing in England. *Arch Dis Child* 89(12):1106–10.

Blair PS, Heron J, Fleming PJ (2010) Relationship between bed sharing and breastfeeding: longitudinal, population-based analysis. *Pediatrics* 126(5):e1119–26.

Blair PS, Sidebotham P, Pease A, Fleming PJ (2014) Bed-sharing in the absence of hazardous circumstances: is there a risk of sudden infant death syndrome? An analysis from two case-control studies conducted in the UK. *PloS One* 9(9):e107799.

Côté A (2006) Bed sharing and sudden infant death syndrome: do we have a definition problem? *Paediatr Child Health* 11(June):34–8.

Crane D, Ball HL (2016) A qualitative study in parental perceptions and understanding of SIDS-reduction guidance in a UK bi-cultural urban community. *BMC Pediatr* 16(1):23.

Crenshaw JT (2014) Healthy birth practice #6: keep mother and baby together – it's best for mother, baby, and breastfeeding. *J Perinatal Educ* 23(4):211–17.

Culver ED (2009) Exploring bed-sharing mothers' motives and decision-making for getting through the night intact: a grounded theory. *J Midwifery Women's Health* 54(5):423.

Doan T, Gardiner A, Gay CL, Lee KA (2007) Breast-feeding increases sleep duration of new parents. *J Perinat Neonat Nursing* 21(3):200–6.

Drever-Smith C, Bogossian F, New K (2013) Co-sleeping and bed sharing in postnatal maternity units: a review of the literature and critique of clinical practice guidelines. *Int J Childbirth* 3(1):13–27.

Elias MF, Nicolson N, Bora C, Johnston J (1986) Sleep/wake patterns of breast-fed infants in the first 2 years of life. *Pediatrics* 77: 322–9.

Feldman-Winter L, Goldsmith JP (2016) Safe sleep and skin-to-skin care in the neonatal period for healthy term newborns. *Pediatrics* 138(3):e20161889.

Fetherston CM, Leach JS (2012) Analysis of the ethical issues in the breastfeeding and bedsharing debate. *Breastfeed Rev* 20(3):7–17.

Galland BC, Taylor BJ, Elder DE, Herbison P (2012) Normal sleep patterns in infants and children: a systematic review of observational studies. *Sleep Med Rev* 16(3):213–22.

Gibson E, Dembofsky CA, Rubin S, Greenspan JS (2000) Infant sleep position practices 2 years into the 'Back to Sleep' campaign. *Clin Pediatr* 39(5):285–9.

Gilbert R, Salanti G, Harden M, See S (2005) Infant sleeping position and the sudden infant death syndrome: systematic review of observational studies and historical review of recommendations from 1940 to 2002. *Int J Epidemiol* 34(4):874–87.

Hardyment C (1983) *Dream Babies*. Oxford: Oxford University Press.

Hauck FR, Signore C, Fein SBSB, Raju TNTNK (2008) Infant sleeping arrangements and practices during the first year of life. *Pediatrics* 122(Supplement 2):S113.

Hauck FR, Thompson JMD, Tanabe KO, Moon RY, Vennemann MM (2011) Breastfeeding and reduced risk of sudden infant death syndrome: a meta-analysis. *Pediatrics* 128(1):103–10.

Henderson JMT, France KG, Owens JL, Blampied NM (2010) Sleeping through the night: the consolidation of self-regulated sleep across the first year of life. *Pediatrics* 126(5):e1081–7.

Horiuchi S, Nishihara K (1999) Analyses of mothers' sleep logs in postpartum periods. *Psychiatry Clin Neurosci* 53(2):137–9.

Howel D, Ball HL (2013) Association between length of exclusive breastfeeding and subsequent breastfeeding continuation. *J Hum Lactat* 29(4):579–85.

Huang Y, Hauck FR, Signore C, Yu A, Raju TNK, Huang TT-K, Fein SB (2013) Influence of bedsharing activity on breastfeeding duration among US mothers. *JAMA Pediatr* 167(11):1038–44.

Joseph D, Chong NW, Shanks ME, Rosato E, Taub NA, Petersen SA, Symonds ME, Whitehouse WP, Wailoo M (2015) Getting rhythm: how do babies do it? *Arch Dis Child – Fetal Neonat Ed* 100(1):F50 LP-F54.

Keefe MR (1988) The impact of infant rooming-in on maternal sleep at night. *J Obstet Gynecol Neonat Nursing: JOGNN* 17(2):122–6.

Kleitman N, Engelmann TG (1953) Sleep characteristics of infants. *J Appl Physiol* 6(5):269–82.

Konner M, Super C (1987) Sudden infant death syndrome: an anthropological hypothesis. In: Super CM (ed.) *The Role of Culture in Developmental Disorder*. San Diego: Academic Press, pp. 95–108.

Lozoff B, Brittenham G (1979) Infant care: cache or carry. *J Pediatr* 95(3):478–83.

Martin RD (2007) The evolution of human reproduction: a primatological perspective. *Yearbook Phys Anthropol* 50:59–84.

McBean AL, Montgomery-Downs HE (2014) What are postpartum women doing while the rest of the world is asleep? *J Sleep Res* 24(3):270–8.

McCoy RC, Hunt CE, Lesko SM, Vezina R, Corwin MJ, Willinger M, Hoffman HJ, Mitchell AA (2004) Frequency of bed sharing and its relationship to breastfeeding. *J Dev Behav Pediatr* 25(3):141–9.

McKenna JJ (1986) An anthropological perspective on the sudden infant death syndrome (SIDS): the role of parental breathing cues and speech breathing adaptations. *Med Anthropol* 10(1):9–92.

McKenna JJ, Gettler LT (2016) There is no such thing as infant sleep, there is no such thing as breastfeeding, there is only breastsleeping. *Acta Paediatr* 105(1):17–21.

McKenna JJ, Thoman EB, Anders TF, Sadeh A, Schechtman VL, Glotzbach SF (1993) Infant–parent co-sleeping in an evolutionary perspective: implications for understanding infant sleep development and the sudden infant death syndrome. *Sleep* 16(3):263–82.

McKenna JJ, Ball HL, Gettler LT (2007) Mother–infant cosleeping, breastfeeding and sudden infant death syndrome: what biological anthropology has discovered about normal infant sleep and pediatric sleep medicine. *Am J Phys Anthropol* 134(S45):133–61.

Mitchell EA, Scragg R (1993) Are infants sharing a bed with another person at increased risk of sudden infant death syndrome? *Sleep* 16(4):387–9.

Montgomery-Downs HE, Clawges HM, Santy EE (2010) Infant feeding methods and maternal sleep and daytime functioning. *Pediatrics* 126(6):e1562–8.

Moon RY, Mathews A, Joyner BL, Oden RP, He J, McCarter R (2017) Health messaging and African-American infant sleep location: a randomized controlled trial. *J Community Health* 42(1):1–9.

Moore T, Ucko LE (1957) Night waking in early infancy: part I. *Arch Dis Child* 32(164):333–42.

Mosko S, Richard C, McKenna J (1997a) Infant arousals during mother–infant bed sharing: implications for infant sleep and sudden infant death syndrome research. *Pediatrics* 100(5):841–9.

Mosko S, Richard C, McKenna J (1997b) Maternal sleep and arousals during bedsharing with infants. *Sleep* 20(2):142–50.

Neville MC (2001) Anatomy and physiology of lactation. *Pediatr Clin North Am* 48(1):13–34.

Neville MC, Morton J (2001) Physiology and endocrine changes underlying human lactogenesis II. *J Nutr* 131(11):3005S–8S.

Parmelee AH, Wenner WH, Schulz HR (1964) Infant sleep patterns: from birth to 16 weeks of age. *J Pediatr* 65(4):576–82.

Quillin SIM, Glenn LL (2004) Interaction between feeding method and co-sleeping on maternal–newborn sleep. *J Obstet Gynecol Neonat Nursing* 33(5):580–8.

Rigda RS, McMillen IC, Buckley P (2000) Bed sharing patterns in a cohort of Australian infants during the first six months after birth. *J Paediatr Child Health* 36(2):117–21.

Riordan J (2011) *Breastfeeding and Human Lactation.* Sudbury, MA: Jones and Bartlett Publishers.

Rudzik AEF, Ball HL (2016) Exploring maternal perceptions of infant sleep and feeding method among mothers in the United Kingdom: a qualitative focus group study. *Matern Child Health J* 20(1):33–40.

Rudzik AEF, Robinson-Smith L, Ball HL (2018) Discrepancies in maternal reports of infant sleep vs. actigraphy by mode of feeding. *Sleep Med* 49:90–8.

Salariya EM, Easton PM, Cater JI (1978) Duration of breast-feeding after early initiation and frequent feeding. *Lancet* 312(8100):1141–3.

Salm Ward TC (2015) Reasons for mother–infant bed-sharing: a systematic narrative synthesis of the literature and implications for future research. *Matern Child Health J* 19(3):675–90.

Santos IS, Mota DM, Matijasevich A, Barros AJD, Barros FCF (2009) Bed-sharing at 3 months and breast-feeding at 1 year in southern Brazil. *J Pediatr* 155(4):505–9.

Scragg RKR, Stewart AW, Mitchell EA, Thompson JMD, Taylor BJBJ, Williams SM … Thompson JMD (1996) Infant room-sharing and prone sleep position in sudden infant death syndrome. *Lancet* 347(8993):7–12.

Tennekoon KH, Arulambalam PD, Karunanayake EH, Seneviratne HR (1994) Prolactin response to suckling in a group of fully breast-feeding women during the early postpartum period. *Asia-Oceania J Obstet Gynaecol* 20(3):311–19.

Thompson JMD, Tanabe K, Moon RY, Mitchell EA, McGarvey C, Tappin D … Hauck FR (2017) Duration of breastfeeding and risk of SIDS: an individual participant data meta-analysis. *Pediatrics* 140(5):e20171324.

Tikotzky L, Marcas G, Har-Toov J, Dollberg S, Bar-Haim Y, Sadeh A (2009) Sleep and physical growth in infants during the first 6 months. *J Sleep Res* 19(1):103–10.

Trevathan WR, Rosenberg K (eds) (2016) *Costly and Cute: Helpless Infants and Human Evolution.* Albuquerque: University of New Mexico Press.

Tully KP, Ball HL (2013) Trade-offs underlying maternal breastfeeding decisions: a conceptual model. *Matern Child Nutr* 9(1):90–8.

Volpe LE, Ball HL, McKenna JJ (2013) Nighttime parenting strategies and sleep-related risks to infants. *Soc Sci Med* 79(1):92–100.

Willinger M, Ko C, Hoffman H (2003) Trends in infant bed sharing in the United States, 1993–2000: the National Infant Sleep Position study. *Arch Pediatr* 157:43–9.

6 Birth experience and breastfeeding

Amy Brown and Jenny Clarke

- Maternal birth experience can have important physiological and psychological impacts upon breastfeeding initiation and continuation. If a mother presents with low milk supply, pain or an infant who has had difficulty latching, ask about her birth experience, both physiological and psychological.
- Mothers who have had a difficult delivery may need additional breastfeeding support in hospital. This might include assistance with holding or moving her infant, help with positioning and attachment and reassurance that her milk may be slightly delayed.
- Skin-to-skin contact after birth helps support breastfeeding for all infants but can be particularly useful if mothers have had a complex delivery or are struggling to express milk for a baby who cannot directly feed.
- For specific information around infant feeding and pain relief or after a caesarean section, see:
  - Pain relief after birth and breastfeeding – www.breastfeeding-and- medication.co.uk/fact-sheet/pain-relief-after-birth-and-breastfeeding
  - Breastfeeding after a caesarean section – https://breastfeedingnetwork. org.uk/wp-content/dibm/Breastfeeding%20after%20a%20caesarean %20section.pdf

Another key influence upon physiological and psychological breastfeeding success is maternal birth experience. Interventions and complications during birth can affect the expected pattern of hormones after the birth, with high levels of the stress hormone cortisol interfering with the hormones needed for breastfeeding – prolactin and oxytocin (Uvnas-Moberg et al. 1990).

Maternal birth experience can also affect the woman psychologically; a mother who feels that her body has let her down or feels traumatised by the birth may find it difficult to believe her body will be able to sustain her baby (Dennis and McQueen 2009). Enabling women to have as normal birth as possible, and recognising the potential impacts of any interventions, is therefore important for breastfeeding success.

Understanding how maternal birth experience can affect breastfeeding is important in supporting women during and after the birth. There are a number of ways in which birth experience can impact upon breastfeeding.

Physiological birth experience

Infants born by caesarean section (particularly emergency section) are less likely to be breastfed (Baxter et al. 2009). Emergency caesarean sections are associated with high levels of maternal cortisol (Grajeda and Pérez-Escamilla 2002) and lower levels of oxytocin and prolactin (Nissen et al. 1995). This pattern of hormones is associated with a lower milk supply, especially if complications mean that the mother did not have immediate skin-to-skin contact with her infant, which can help raise oxytocin levels (Bystrova et al. 2003).

Infants born by caesarean section can have altered feeding behaviours. Tongue movement is subdued, whilst suck is often faster and harder in an attempt to remove milk. This can lead to a less effective milk transfer, pain in the mother and as a consequence lower milk supply (Sakalidis et al. 2013). Infants born by assisted delivery can also have an increased risk of latching difficulties and are less likely to be breastfed by 2 weeks (Brown and Jordan 2013). This is likely due to soreness or even damage to their head area (Wall and Glass 2006), as well as the impact of high cortisol levels in the mother during a difficult birth (Nissen et al. 1995).

Further complications during and after the birth can also affect milk supply. Postpartum haemorrhage (PPH), induction and augmentation of birth and fetal distress are associated with increased breastfeeding difficulties and cessation (Brown and Jordan 2013). A PPH is associated with lower prolactin levels due to a drop in blood pressure, which can affect milk production (Willis and Livingstone 1995). Synthetic oxytocin is often used to induce or accelerate birth, or as PPH treatment. However evidence suggests it might reduce maternal natural prolactin and oxytocin production, impacting on milk supply (Jonas et al. 2009).

Pain relief used during labour and birth

There are a number of studies that have identified a link between pain relief during labour and subsequent infant feeding behaviours. Pethidine is recognised as subduing the infant, leading to decreased rooting for the nipple, a weaker suck and a poorer latch (Nissen et al. 1996). Epidurals have also been linked to a shorter breastfeeding duration, partly but independently from their association with caesarean birth (Jordan 2005). Mothers who have an epidural have lower levels of oxytocin after the birth (Goodfellow et al. 1983). It is thought that the anaesthetic blocks feeling of the Ferguson reflex, which is associated with oxytocin release (Levy et al. 1992).

In each of these scenarios, mothers who have had interventions or complications during childbirth are more likely to be experiencing residual pain and reduced mobility after the birth. They may be separated from their infant or less likely to have skin-to-skin contact. All of these mean that infants may feed less frequently, with a reduction in milk supply as a consequence.

Psychological impact

Maternal birth experience can affect how she feels about her body and the confidence she has to breastfeed. A difficult birth is associated with increased risk of anxiety, depression and birth trauma which in turn are associated with lower levels of breastfeeding (Simpson and Catling 2016). Psychological experience of childbirth can also affect breastfeeding by reducing maternal confidence in her body (Beck and Watson 2008). She may feel that if her body 'didn't work' during labour, why would it work to feed her baby?

The benefits of skin-to-skin contact after the birth

Humans are born expecting to be held and touched by their mother. Skin-to-skin contact is the grand finale to pregnancy and a building block of the synergistic relationship between a mother and her child. Early skin-to-skin contact means an improvement in two-way dyad attachment behaviour (Moore et al. 2016). A midwife's role is to facilitate this quietly and efficiently by supporting the mother to embrace her newborn as immediately as possible after birth. In supporting the integrity of the dyad, the midwife is acting on her or his understanding of psychological, social, emotional and spiritual factors that may positively or adversely influence normal physiology, and displaying competency in this practice (Nursing & Midwifery Council 2018).

The research and evidence show that the effects that skin-to-skin contact can have on a mother and her newborn are more than physiological. Crenshaw (2007) found that in minimising separation we can reduce the chances of harm from inadequate care later. Skin-to-skin contact also has an effect on the reciprocal relationship between the mother and her child. Newborns who had skin-to-skin contact, suckling and/or both displayed a positive interaction 1 year after birth with their mothers compared to those having no skin to skin. Thus, when a mother embraces her newborn infant immediately after birth in skin-to-skin contact, it has a profound impact on her self-belief, mood and wellbeing.

A review of mothers' experiences of skin-to-skin contact discovered that women felt overwhelming love, an instinctive ability to mother their child, a positive feeling of self-esteem and an ability to understand their child (Moore et al. 2016). Skin to skin also boosts the production of maternal oxytocin, helping both the uterus to contract and also vasodilatation of vessels on the skin of the abdomen and chest, therefore protecting the baby from the adverse effects of hypothermia and hypoglycaemia when in skin to skin (Bystrova et al. 2003). Maintaining the temperature of a term baby through skin to skin is key to preventing admission to the neonatal unit (ATAIN study 2017) and it's great to see campaigns sparked by this on Twitter from maternity units in the UK to promote skin-to-skin contact in all birth settings.

Within my own practice (Jenny Clarke) I have supported women with skin to skin in various emergency situations and received feedback that the act of skin to skin has taken the woman's mind away from her own fear. Dr Diane Ménage's Doctoral research involved extensive interviews with women who said they had experienced compassionate midwifery care (Ménage 2019). The women in the research made it clear that compassionate care helped them with fear, feeling vulnerable, feeling out of control and having a lack of knowledge. Compassionate midwifery is an intervention which increases trust and makes a profound difference to women. Facilitating skin-to-skin contact is therefore an act of compassionate midwifery which supports both members of the dyad.

Yet many mothers and babies are still not receiving this opportunity. In the foreword of *Impact of Birthing Practices on Breastfeeding* (Smith and Kroeger 2010), Dr Nils Bergman writes, 'almost everything we do to try and improve on the self-sustaining dyad is detrimental to mother and baby', yet how often is skin-to-skin contact recognised as both normal and important for mother and baby? Do we question the long- and short-term impact of maternal infant separation with the same passion with which we celebrate the benefits of skin-to-skin contact success?

Maternal pain medication after the birth

It is important that maternal pain is well controlled after birth, particularly if the birth was a caesarean section or instrumental delivery. One of the most important factors in achieving effective positioning and attachment is that the mother is able to sit, lie and move comfortably, which is impossible if she is in unrelenting pain. When it was first recommended that codeine was no longer to be prescribed during lactation, many clinicians struggled to be confident in prescribing an alternative. There were anecdotal reports on social media of mothers being denied anything more than paracetamol and ibuprofen regardless of reported pain. This unsurprisingly led to mothers feeling that they had no option but to formula-feed, at least temporarily. Hospital guidelines now routinely use paracetamol plus a non-steroidal anti-inflammatory (ibuprofen, diclofenac or naproxen) and as required Oramorph and/or dihydrocodeine. Most discharge prescriptions are for diclofenac/naproxen with dihydrocodeine/co-dydramol for up to a week after delivery. These drugs are all compatible with breastfeeding (Jones 2018).

Postnatal environment

The environment on the postnatal ward can also affect a mother's breastfeeding success. Mothers who birth in a UNICEF Baby Friendly-accredited hospital where steps are taken to protect breastfeeding are more likely to breastfeed; such steps include providing education, expert support and ensuring mother and baby are kept together where possible. The more steps a hospital adheres to, the better the breastfeeding outcomes. Although each step is important, community-based support on discharge has been shown to have the most impact (Perez-Escamilla et al. 2016).

If an infant needs to go to neonatal intensive care

Breastmilk is important for all infants but particularly vital for premature infants. However, the more premature the infant, the more difficult establishing breastfeeding can be (Vohr et al. 2007). Infants born prior to 34 weeks can experience latch difficulties as their sucking reflex is not yet fully developed (Nyqvist et al. 1999). Mothers often need to express milk, which can be challenging in a stressful environment. Stress itself should not affect milk production, but it can affect the milk ejection reflex, meaning mothers find it more difficult to get a let-down, increasing concerns around milk supply (Dewey 2001). Skin-to-skin contact would support this, including holding their infant if fed through a tube. However, mothers can worry about their tiny, fragile-looking infant (Flacking et al. 2007).

In summary, maternal birth experience can play an important physiological and psychological role in affecting her ability to breastfeed. If a mother presents with low milk supply or an infant who cannot latch comfortably, take a full birth history. If working with mothers in hospital settings, remember that protecting the birth environment to reduce complications can help support breastfeeding. Mothers who have a difficult birth may need further support postnatally to establish breastfeeding.

References

ATAIN study (2017) *NHS Improvement. Reducing Harm Leading to Avoidable Admission of Full-Term Babies to Neonatal Units.* London: NHS Improvement.

Baxter J, Cooklin AR, Smith J (2009) Which mothers wean their babies prematurely from full breastfeeding? An Australian cohort study. *Acta Paediatr* 98(8):1274–7.

Beck CT, Watson S (2008) Impact of birth trauma on breast-feeding: a tale of two pathways. *Nurs Res* 57(4):228–36.

Brown A, Jordan S (2013) Impact of birth complications on breastfeeding duration: an Internet survey. *J Adv Nurs* 69(4):828–39.

Bystrova K, Widström AM, Matthiesen AS (2003) Skin-to-skin contact may reduce negative consequences of "the stress of being born": a study on temperature in new-born infants, subjected to different ward routines in St Petersburg. *Acta Paediatr* 92(3):320–6.

Crenshaw JT (2007) Care practice #6: no separation of mother and baby, with unlimited opportunities for breastfeeding. *J Perinat Educ Summer* 16(3):39–43.

Dennis CL, McQueen K (2009) The relationship between infant-feeding outcomes and postpartum depression: a qualitative systematic review. *Pediatrics* 123(4):e736–51.

Dewey KG (2001) Maternal and fetal stress are associated with impaired lactogenesis in humans. *J Nutr* 131(11):3012S–15S.

Flacking R, Ewald U, Starrin B (2007) "I wanted to do a good job": experiences of 'becoming a mother' and breastfeeding in mothers of very preterm infants after discharge from a neonatal unit. *Soc Sci Med* 64(12):2405–16.

Goodfellow CF, Hull MGR, Swaab DF (1983) Oxytocin deficiency at delivery with epidural analgesia. *BJOG* 90(3):214–19.

Grajeda R, Pérez-Escamilla R (2002) Stress during labor and delivery is associated with delayed onset of lactation among urban Guatemalan women. *J Nutr* 132(10):3055–60.

Jonas W, Johansson LM, Nissen E (2009) Effects of intrapartum oxytocin administration and epidural analgesia on the concentration of plasma oxytocin and prolactin, in response to suckling during the second day postpartum. *Breastfeed Med* 4(2):71–82.

Jones, W (2018) *Breastfeeding and Medication.* London: Routledge.

Jordan S, Emery S, Bradshaw C (2005) The impact of intrapartum analgesia on infant feeding. *BJOG* 112(7):927–34.

Levy F, Kendrick KM, Keverne EB (1992) Intracerebral oxytocin is important for the onset of maternal behavior in inexperienced ewes delivered under peridural anesthesia. *Behav Neurosci* 106:427–32.

Menage D (2019) Women's lived-experience of compassionate midwifery. Unpublished thesis. Coventry University, UK.

Moore ER, Bergman N, Anderson GC, Medley N (2016) Early skin to skin contact for mothers and their healthy newborn infants. *Cochrane Database System Rev.*

Nissen E, Lilja G, Matthiesen AS (1995) Effects of maternal pethidine on infants' developing breast feeding behaviour. *Acta Paediatr* 84(2):140–5.

Nissen E, Uvnäs-Moberg K, Svensson K (1996) Different patterns of oxytocin, prolactin but not cortisol release during breastfeeding in women delivered by caesarean section or by the vaginal route. *Early Hum Dev* 45(1–2):103–18.

Nursing & Midwifery Council (2018) The Code: Standards for Competence for Registered Midwives. www.nmc.org.uk/standards/standards-for-midwives/standards-of-competence-for-registered-midwives/

Nyqvist KH, Sjödén PO, Ewald U (1999) The development of preterm infants' breastfeeding behavior. *Early Hum Dev* 55(3):247–64.

Pérez-Escamilla R, Martinez JL, Segura-Pérez S (2016) Impact of the Baby-friendly Hospital Initiative on breastfeeding and child health outcomes: a systematic review. *Matern Child Nutr* 12(3):402–17.

Sakalidis VS, Williams TM, Hepworth AR (2013) A comparison of early sucking dynamics during breastfeeding after cesarean section and vaginal birth. *Breastfeed Med* 8(1):79–85.

Simpson M, Catling C (2016) Understanding psychological traumatic birth experiences: a literature review. *Women Birth* 29(3):203–7.

Smith LJ, Kroeger M (2010) Impact of *Birthing Practices* on *Breastfeeding*. Jones & Bartlett Publishers.Uvnäs-Moberg K, Widström AM, Werner S (1990) Oxytocin and prolactin levels in breast-feeding women. Correlation with milk yield and duration of breast-feeding. *Acta Obstet Gynecol Scand* 69(4):301–6.

Vohr BR, Poindexter BB, Dusick AM (2007) Persistent beneficial effects of breast milk ingested in the neonatal intensive care unit on outcomes of extremely low birth weight infants at 30 months of age. *Pediatrics* 120(4):e953–9.

Wall V, Glass R (2006) Mandibular asymmetry and breastfeeding problems: experience from 11 cases. *J Hum Lactat* 22(3):328–34.

Willis CE, Livingstone V (1995) Infant insufficient milk syndrome associated with maternal postpartum hemorrhage. *J Hum Lactat* 11(2):123–6.

7 Breastfeeding complications

Emma Pickett and Wendy Jones

- Many new families we support will have little experience of breastfeeding and may only see a baby breastfeed up close for the first time when they come to feed their own baby.
- Babies are surprisingly able when it comes to attaching to the breast and baby-led attachment is increasingly encouraged.
- When mothers do guide the baby, there are some key principles that can make breastfeeding a comfortable and effective process.
- A lack of familiarity with normal newborn behaviour can also bring some challenges. Families benefit from understanding that breastfeeding is more than a milk delivery system and comfort, aiding sleep and relationship-building are all to be valued.
- A newborn baby may breastfeed more frequently than families might expect, especially when older relatives are recalling guidelines from previous decades.
- A newborn baby feeding frequently is aiding the development of milk supply, preventing engorgement, blocked ducts and mastitis and setting up a scenario where a family are more likely to reach their breastfeeding goals.

Breastfeeding may be natural but just like many physical skills it is a learning process that happens over time between mother and baby. There are a number of key elements around recognising when breastfeeding is going well, and when complications are arising, that will help mothers continue to breastfeed for longer. Central to this is the concept of positioning and attachment, or how the infant latches on to the breast. If this step is not well supported, the risk of a number of complications can arise.

Positioning and attachment

Effective positioning and attachment of the baby at the breast are at the heart of successful breastfeeding (Figure 7.1). If a mother is experiencing difficulties, it is appropriate to signpost to local breastfeeding support. This will vary across the country but should include the opportunity for face-to-face support with someone trained in breastfeeding most days of the week. However, it is useful if medical professionals are familiar with some of the basic principles. The acronym CHINS is often used.

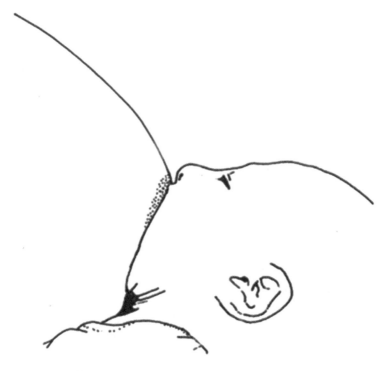

Figure 7.1 Effective latch
Source: ©Jennifer N Richardson from a photograph by Nancy Durrell McKenna.

- The baby is *close* with *head free* (the head is able to tilt back and supported around the shoulders and neck only). The head will tilt as the baby comes to the breast so the chin leads.
- The baby is *in line* (so the neck isn't twisted while attempting to swallow).
- Mothers are often told *nose* to *nipple* so that the nipple is above the baby's top lip to maximise the head tilt and the chin coming to the breast. As the baby opens the mouth wide, the nipple is extended towards the junction of the hard and soft palate.
- The position needs to be *sustainable* so the mother has whole-body comfort, does not feel her arms, hands and back are taking strain and the baby can maintain the position (www.wirralct.nhs.uk/you-and-your-health/healthy-living/breastfeeding/how-to).

There is not one standard breastfeeding position that works for all. Some of the traditional positions where a mother is advised to sit upright with a breastfeeding pillow can cause significant complications. Factors like the fall of the breasts, the angle of the nipple, the gap between breast and lap and the length of a mother's arm bones will all mean an individualised position is needed. Increasingly, mothers are being encouraged to recline either for the first breastfeed or as the baby grows (https://midwiferytoday.com/mt-articles/biological-nurturing/). Baby-led attachment is often

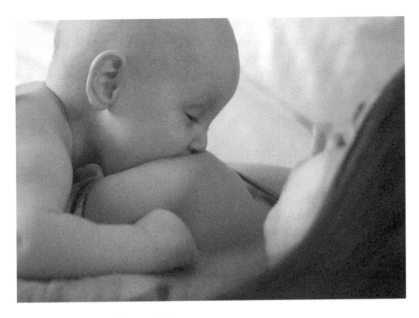

Figure 7.2 Reclined breastfeeding
Source: Shutterstock image.

effective. Ideally, a mother will not be holding or manipulating her breast. A baby can breathe even with a nose that is making contact with a large soft breast, due to nostril shape, and it is not necessary for a breast to be pushed out of the way with a finger which may be utilised better elsewhere (including feeding and watering the mother). Babies will prioritise breathing, which is why they should be given the flexibility to move their head. Learning to feed while lying down is also a skill many mothers come to value as it enables them to rest and even sleep while baby is feeding (Figure 7.2).

When positioning is not ideal, feeds may be longer and uncomfortable. The baby may ingest more air, become unsettled and may be at risk of insufficient intake. The mother risks nipple damage, blocked ducts, mastitis and supply problems.

Engorgement

Postpartum engorgement is common for mothers at around day 2–5. As the interstitial fluid, blood and milk accumulate, the mother will experience fullness and often some discomfort. As the breast tissue tightens and the nipple may appear flatter, latching can become temporarily more challenging. Mothers can be shown how to use 'reverse pressure softening' to move fluid away from the areola and nipple (Cotterman 2004). Cold compresses will also promote lymph drainage and a mother can massage towards the armpit to speed up this process. Hand expression may make latching a little easier but excessive pumping may complicate messages to her supply. In severe cases, ibuprofen may be used. If a baby is latching effectively and frequently from the start, engorgement may be eased. There is also research that suggests mothers who receive intravenous fluid in labour are more likely to experience complications with breast engorgement (Berens and Brodribb 2016).

After the postpartum phase, engorgement may recur as the baby's patterns adjust or sometimes in response to an artificial gap between feeds. Mothers benefit from understanding the link between engorgement and an increased risk of blocked ducts and mastitis, but also from an appreciation that engorgement is a natural process which enables the breasts to match a baby's new routines and sends signals to adjust supply, e.g. breasts feeling temporarily fuller when baby starts sleeping for longer blocks at night.

Nipple pain

Nipple pain should not be considered an accepted part of normal breastfeeding and pain requires investigation to prevent early weaning (Kent et al. 2015). However, even when the baby's attachment is optimum, there may be some discomfort during the initial latch for the first few days. In these circumstances, the nipple should exit baby's mouth extended but rounded at the end rather than wedge-shaped, with a white compression stripe or flattened. The discomfort should ease once active feeding begins after around the first 20–30 seconds.

If the nipple is exiting the baby's mouth *flattened, misshapen to a point or with a compression stripe*, or if the mother is in pain throughout a feed, adjusting the latch should be the first consideration. When a nipple is sitting correctly in space around the junction of the hard and soft palate, there is nothing to misshape it. When positioning and attachment are problematic, the nipple may start to become damaged by abrasion against the palate, rear of the tongue or by a baby overcompensating for an ineffective latch with a stronger suck. The situation can often be corrected by even small adjustments to the baby's position and ensuring the baby is well supported at the breast. Compression from a less than optimum attachment can result in vasospasm and deep breast pain after a feed.

Adjustments may include bringing the baby's chin and upper body closer to the breast and encouraging the baby to tilt the head on approach to the breast so that the chin comes away from the chest. It can be helpful to remind parents that when we drink from a glass of water, we naturally lift our chin and we want the baby to have the opportunity to do the same.

It may be that the baby's body needs greater support so that s/he feels more anchored and gravity is not pulling on a mother's arms and hands which may drift during a feed. If the mother is sitting upright, does the baby start at a height where their nose is naturally level with the nipple and does the baby comfortably remain at that height? Is the baby's arm trapped between the baby's body and the breast or is clothing bunching up and moving the baby away from the mother's body? If a mother is struggling with pain during feeds, introducing a more reclined position may be helpful.

A nipple that is compressed by less than ideal latching may look *white at the end of a feed* due to vasospasm. This can mean pain during a feed and afterwards as the blood flow returns. Correcting the latch will ultimately alleviate the problem but applying dry heat immediately after a feed may also help.

If the latching appears good and *the nipple is not misshaping, but there is still whiteness and particularly discomfort* after a feed, *circulation issues* may be the cause. Mothers with Raynaud's syndrome may find the discomfort at the end of a feed particularly challenging and a triphasic colour change may be seen (white, blue, before returning to red if a nipple was initially pinky red). Use of nifedipine is compatible with breastfeeding (www.wirralct.nhs.uk/you-and-your-health/healthy-living/breastfeeding/how-to).

Raynaud's phenomenon is characterised by:

- pain which worsens in the cold, e.g. passing fridges in the supermarket or even exposure of the nipple to feed;
- bi- or triphasic colour changes immediately after feeds;
- history of circulation problems or close family history of circulation problems;
- history of migraines;
- early delivery of baby or small baby – due to vasoconstriction of placental blood vessels.

Self-help treatment includes ensuring that any problems with the latch have been dealt with and applying warm heat to the breasts immediately after a feed, e.g. use of a warm wheat bag. Sources have suggested the use of ginger, high doses of vitamin B_6, magnesium, calcium, fatty acids and fish oil supplementation but these take a minimum of 6 weeks to be effective. Treatment with nifedipine 10 mg three times a day or long-acting formulation 30 mg once a day is effective and safe in breastfeeding as little passes into milk.

If a mother has a *cracked nipple*, resolving the underlying cause is obviously the priority. In the meantime, evidence suggests that the use of nipple creams does not promote faster healing or relieve pain (Jackson and Watson 2014). Applying breastmilk or nothing may be just as beneficial according to the Cochrane review (www.cochrane.org/CD007366/PREG_interventions-for-treating-painful-nipples-among-breastfeeding-women).

When the *damage is deeper*, moist wound healing is considered good practice. Although mothers are likely to have received the message that certain products are superior, soft white paraffin, hydrogel dressings and lanolin all seem to prevent the formation of a scab and promote faster healing equally well and research is inconclusive as to which method is preferable.

When a *nipple is itchy*, an allergy should be considered which may be triggered by exposure to a new product or material, e.g. exposure to breast pads. A low-dose topical steroid applied sparingly after feeds may help. However, the cause of discomfort may be related to breastfeeding technique, so face-to-face support with a specialist may be recommended.

If a mother is *still in pain* despite her nipple not misshaping and after she has received qualified support in positioning and attachment, an *infection* may be suspected. There may be a history of latching problems as damage caused from positioning has increased the risk of infection, but infection will present with some key features.

A *bacterial infection* (commonly *Staphylococcus aureus*) will often present with a yellow discharge and the nipple shows signs of redness and irritation. It will usually be limited to one side and there is no risk to the baby if breastfeeding continues as normal. A topical antibiotic treatment which contains hydrocortisone may be appropriate.

Bacterial and fungal infections on the nipple can be identified with a swab. *Thrush* on the nipple is more likely when either member of the dyad has had recent antibiotics. The nipple often appears scaly or shiny and is sensitive to any touch. Mothers who have pink nipples may notice the nipple is redder than usual. Mothers with darker skin may notice a loss of pigment on the areola, though this can occur with any mother. If a nipple is temporarily paler or white during a feed, this would indicate compression or vasospasm rather than thrush.

Thrush will transfer quickly to both nipples so, if only one nipple is affected, a bacterial infection or a complication with latching should be considered. Nipple thrush can result in deeper breast pain from neuralgia. In the past, deep breast pain was sometimes described as ductal thrush. Evidence as to whether *Candida* can colonise the milk ducts is lacking but oral antifungal medication is often effective with some considerations. When thrush is suspected, both mother and baby will need treatment, even in the absence of one member of the dyad having symptoms.

Symptoms of thrush are:

- painful nipples after feeds;
- white tongue in the baby;
- pain lasting for up to an hour after feeds;
- pain in both breasts after every feed;
- positive swabs of the mother's nipples and baby's mouth

Candidiasis should not be diagnosed where the feeds themselves are painful, where the tip of the nipple is white after feeds, or shaped/flattened, where the pain is described as pinpoint with a white spot on the nipple visible or where there are cracks which may have a bacterial infection. Symptoms can be mistaken for vasospasm (treated by attention to optimising position and attachment supported by a lactation expert) and Raynaud's phenomenon.

Optimal treatment for the baby is miconazole oral gel applied gently a small amount at a time until all surfaces of the tongue are coated four times a day. Although the licence states that it should not be used in babies under 4 months, this is due to the risk of the method of application rather than the drug itself (Ainsworth and Jones 2009). It should not be applied to the mother's nipples as a means of covering the baby's tongue as this may lead to choking. Nystatin suspension is only fungistatic and not fungicidal and achieves only a cure of 54% in 10 days, compared to 99% with miconazole (Hoppe and Hahn 1996; Hoppe 1997).

The mother should apply miconazole cream sparingly to her nipples after every feed and not wash it off to avoid further damage. Clotrimazole is less effective and appears anecdotally to cause allergic reactions (Jones 2018).

If symptoms persist despite topical treatment and attention to positioning and attachment, the prescription of fluconazole 150–400 mg as a starting dose followed by 100–200 mg daily for 7–10 days may be necessary. Caution should be exercised if the baby is less than 6 weeks as fluconazole has an extended half-life in neonates. Accumulation may lead to vomiting, weight loss and stomach cramps (Jones 2018, personal communication). If resolution does not occur in 10 days reconsider the diagnosis.

Breast pain

Any discomfort at the nipple, whether from infection or attachment, can result in deeper breast pain. Referred pain may even be experienced in the shoulders or back.

Mothers may be unaware than the milk ejection reflex (or 'let-down') can result in some sharp pains at the start of a feed. This usually becomes less severe over time.

Blocked duct

When milk is not removed effectively, a mother may develop a blocked duct. This term may refer to an actual blockage in a milk duct or insufficient milk removal, resulting in a localised immune response from overly full glandular tissue. Risk factors include tight clothing, a hand pressing into the breast or a shallow latch from positioning and attachment issues. Frequent milk removal with improved positioning, massage and warm compresses can alleviate symptoms.

Bleb/white spot

A blocked duct may also present on the nipple at the duct ending and is described as a 'bleb' or milk blister. Milk flow may return after the blister has been pierced with a sterile needle and the breast compressed to remove any hardened material.

Mastitis

Firmness from a blocked duct can develop into non-infective mastitis and then, subsequently, infective mastitis. Infective mastitis may develop suddenly, especially when nipple damage allows an entry point for bacteria. Mastitis is a relatively common condition, affecting up to 20% of lactating women, and the risk is higher in the first 6 weeks (Amir 2014). The breast is likely to be red, although this will not be an identifying feature in mothers with dark skin. The breast will contain a firm lump or wedge alongside the inflammation and the mother will present with a temperature exceeding 38.5°C. A fissure may show signs of *S. aureus* infection. She may have flu-like symptoms and chills.

In most cases mastitis is an inflammatory response and does not require immediate prescription of antibiotics. Frequent, effective milk removal together with the use of ibuprofen may be sufficient. Research shows that, even with antibiotic treatment, resolution of symptoms is more rapid if accompanied by help to remove milk optimally (Thomsen et al. 1984). If the mother is clinically unwell the World Health Organization (WHO) (2000) recommendation is prescription of flucloxacillin 250–500 mg four times a day or amoxicillin 250–500 mg three times a day or, in the case of penicillin allergy, erythromycin 250–500 mg four times a day or cephalexin 250–500 mg four times a day. Frequent milk removal should continue throughout the treatment period and breastfeeding does not need to be interrupted (Amir 2014).

In the absence of sepsis or other complications, a mother can be treated with antibiotics at home alongside continued breastfeeding and milk removal.

Abscess

In about 3% of women with mastitis, the firm area in the breast remains and an abscess which will not respond to antibiotic treatment is suspected. Needle aspiration under ultrasound guidance is commonly used and may be repeated more than once. Dealing with an abscess does not mean an interruption to breastfeeding, although the mother may need support finding a comfortable position.

Non-attachment/breast rejection

The last national infant feeding survey revealed that, of the women who gave up breastfeeding in the first 2 weeks postpartum, a third did so because of the baby's rejection of the breast. Breast refusal is rarely discussed antenatally and often has a significant emotional impact on new parents. It happens for a variety of reasons: some connected to the physiology of the baby but more commonly affected by birth experience (Smith 2007).

An initial delay after an assisted delivery may have a short-lived effect but may impact on maternal confidence as well as the ability to do some effective early feeds. As feeding is less frequent or effective, the mother's engorgement can become a further barrier to milk removal and the situation is further complicated.

Sometimes what is perceived as a baby's refusal to breastfeed is in fact related to positioning and attachment issues. A mother (or someone trying to assist her) may be forcefully holding a baby's head which triggers a reflex to pull back further or a baby may not be close enough to the breast and the necessary triggers for a successful feed are not being stimulated.

When babies are not feeding directly at the breast, parents may become engaged in lengthy attempts to encourage a latch. This could result in baby feeding insufficiently and a mother's milk supply not receiving necessary stimulation. They should be directed to prioritise skin-to-skin contact, feeding the baby, protecting supply and then working on the breastfeeding. This may mean shorter breastfeeding sessions followed by feeding from a cup or syringe, expressing both breasts and keeping mother and baby close. The breastfeeding attempt may also be more positive if the baby has already received some other milk.

In the first 2–3 days, mothers can be supported to hand express initially and catch colostrum drips with a syringe. They may then use an electric breast pump for additional stimulation. When babies are born prematurely and are non-attaching, a mother will be directed to begin expressing within 6 hours of birth. She then continues to express approximately eight times in 24 hours with an acknowledgement that overnight pumping is essential to take advantage of the prolactin hormone's natural circadian rhythms. Hands-on pumping is known to increase output (Morton et al. 2009).

Nipple shields can be a tool used with guidance, but there may be negative consequences (Chow et al. 2015). If shields are to be used, the modern silicone options appear to have a less detrimental impact on milk supply than shields manufactured from firmer material. Shields should be sized according to the diameter of the base of the mother's nipple (small (16 mm), medium (20 mm) and large (24 mm) are readily available in the UK). Sizing is according to mother's anatomy, rather than baby's. The shield can also be applied slightly inside-out to create negative pressure when the shield is reinverted, allowing a tight fit and the nipple to be extended further inside the barrel of the shield.

Low milk supply/perceptions of low milk supply

Concerns about low milk supply affect almost all new families at some point. When breastfeeding is a new experience and newborn behaviour and milk production may not be fully understood, the tendency to doubt milk supply is common.

This may sometimes be justified, as will be indicated by weight gain issues or insufficient stooling and urine output. In rare cases, the cause may be breast hypoplasia. Estimates suggest 1–5% of the population may have 'insufficient glandular tissue', although the use of this term with mothers is problematic (Neifert et al. 1985). These mothers may have experienced little breast changes in puberty and pregnancy. Breasts may be widely spaced, asymmetrical or tubular in appearance with a bulging proportionately large areola. Attempting to diagnose hypoplasia of the breast based on appearance is unreliable. The mother may have had little sense of postpartum engorgement. Baby may not be audibly swallowing and is likely to require supplementation at an early stage.

In approximately one-third of women with polycystic ovary syndrome, low milk supply may also be an issue (Kirigin Bilos 2017). Increase in milk supply may be assisted by use of metformin. Other risk factors include significant blood loss, fragments of retained placenta (Anderson 2001), breast surgery, thyroid dysfunction (Stuebe 2015) and insulin resistance (Nommsen-Rivers 2016).

In cases with primary lactation challenges, mothers can be reassured that efforts to maximise the amount of breast milk given are worthwhile and even small amounts of breastmilk can be beneficial. Supply will be improved with increased milk removal, which will include feeding the baby responsively and encouraging frequent feeding, not restricting the baby to feeding only at one breast for each feed (this can include using each breast several times, known as 'switch nursing') and ensuring the baby's positioning and attachment are as efficient as possible.

Sometimes a mother may be encouraged to use a breast pump in addition to feeding directly at the breast. Hospital-grade double pumps can be rented to help make the pumping sessions more time-efficient and mothers can use hands-on pumping techniques to increase output, which includes breast massage prior to pumping, compressing and massaging during the main pumping session and hand expression afterwards.

Mothers may choose to use a supplementary nutritional system directly at the breast, using a tube to deliver additional milk as a baby breastfeeds. This increases breast stimulation, reinforces the baby's abilities at the breast and can give both mother and baby a sense of closeness that is a valued aspect of breastfeeding.

In some cases, a mother may be considered for a galactagogue. These are commonly herbal but a mother may not always be aware of the contraindications of a commonly used galactagogue like fenugreek (which may interfere with thyroid function or have implications for mothers with asthma or blood sugar disorders). Domperidone and metoclopramide are also used in the UK and around the world with certain reservations.

You are likely to encounter few mothers with primary lactation challenges but more with secondary issues due to insufficient milk removal. Difficulties with positioning and attachment will lead to less efficient signals to the drive to build milk production. A longer feed may not be a more effective one. The link between frequent and efficient milk removal and milk supply is not always appreciated. Families may incorrectly perceive that the breasts need to 'fill' or that feeding or pumping frequently may deprive the baby of volume or quality of milk. Attempting to implement a feeding schedule, restricting time at the breast (perhaps with a misunderstanding that babies should be removed after X number of minutes and moved to the other side) and the use of supplements and artificial nipples may all lead to a decreased milk supply. As mothers' confidence fades and more supplementation is used, the supply can decrease further.

Perceptions of low milk supply are widespread in a culture where newborn baby behaviour is not always well understood. The 20th-century misperception that feeding after 3 or 4 hours is the norm for a newborn has led to much confusion and frequent confidence issues· A normal newborn cluster feeding for a continuous period of 3 or more hours, waking frequently, desiring to be held close and to spend time comforting him- or herself on the breast may be wrongly perceived as an indication of milk supply problems. Even when weight gain and urine and stool output suggest otherwise, parents may doubt milk production and have their confidence further knocked when other natural processes occur: a mother no longer sensing the milk ejection ('let-down') reflex, a mother no longer leaking or feeling engorgement between feeds, a mother who doesn't easily elicit a milk ejection reflex when using a breast pump.

With both perceptions of low milk supply and actual low milk supply, a breastfeeding peer support network with signposting opportunities to specialist services such as an International Board Certified Lactation Consultant (IBCLC) will be valuable.

Oversupply

While many mothers are concerned about insufficient milk supply, an overproduction of breastmilk can bring significant challenges. It isn't clear why some mothers produce more milk than is a required, although the widespread use of electric breast pumps in the early stages of lactation may be a contributing factor. Signs will include a baby struggling with flow at the breast, spluttering, coming off and reluctant to return. Baby is likely to be exceeding normal weight gain expectations and the mother will often feel overly full and uncomfortable. Babies may show signs of digestive discomfort which can be related to ingesting air as they try and coordinate their breathing pattern in the face of a faster flow (or 'overactive let-down'). Symptoms that are sometimes described as 'colic' may also be related to ingesting more lactose than can be digested, despite normal lactase production. This can result in faster gut transit and green, sometimes frothy, stools. This is sometimes confused with a dairy allergy or other food intolerance (Woolridge and Fisher 1988).

There is some suggestion that dyads struggling with oversupply may not see excessive weight gain, but instead have a baby taking proportionally less of the fattier milk at the end of the feed and instead feeding frequently on the earlier lower-fat content milk. However great care needs to be taken where a baby struggling with oversupply is gaining weight insufficiently as the issues may be a baby struggling with flow for other reasons – some physiological, others related to latch – rather than because of overproduction.

When overproduction is clear, a mother can be supported to manage her use of expressing to reduce breast stimulation. She may be automatically offering both breasts at one feed while the baby may be sufficiently satisfied with only one. By leaving the other breast at maximum storage capacity, it is thought it will accumulate a whey protein 'feedback inhibitor of lactation' and the prolactin receptors will be distended, which will reduce messages to stimulate production. A further stage is known as 'block nursing', where one breast is left unused for a longer period of time (initially 4–6 hours) (van Veldhuizen-Staas 2007).

This needs to be managed carefully as a mother may be at greater risk of blocked ducts and mastitis and this is a group already likely to be at higher risk of breast problems.

Summary

Effective positioning and attachment at the breast are key to preventing a wide range of breastfeeding problems: soreness, nipple damage, infection risk, an unsettled baby, insufficient milk transfer and weight gain problems. Once issues are resolved, milk supply can increase again at any stage of breastfeeding by increasing the frequency of feeding or pumping.

Even a short consultation can identify key problems with attachment. Is the mother's nipple squashed on exit from the breast? Is she lifting the breast towards the baby rather than moving the baby to her? Is the baby taking a wide mouthful of breast with rounded cheeks and chin contact? National helplines such as the National Breastfeeding Helpline (0300 100 0212) and the National Childbirth Trust (NCT) feeding line (0300 330 0700) can provide support, although ideally the mother should be able to access a face-to-face breastfeeding group.

References

Ainsworth S, Jones W (2009) It sticks in our throats too. *BMJ* 338:3178.

Amir LH (2014) ABM clinical protocol #4: mastitis. *Breastfeed Med* 9(5).

Anderson AM (2001) Disruption of lactogenesis by retained placental fragments. *J Hum Lactat* 17(2):142–4.

Berens P, Brodribb W (2016) ABM clinical protocol #20: engorgement, revised 2016. *Breastfeed Med* 11(4):159–63.

Chow S, Popovic M, Lam H, Merrick J, Ventegodt S, Milakovic M, Lam M, Popovic M, Chow E, Popovic J (2015) The use of nipple shields: a review. *Front Public Health* 3:236.

Cotterman K (2004) Reverse pressure softening: a simple tool to prepare areola for easier latching during engorgement. *J Hum Lactat* 20(2):227–37.

Hoppe JE, Hahn H (1996) Randomized comparison of two nystatin oral gels with miconazole oral gel for treatment of oral thrush in infants. *Infection* 24(2):136–9.

Hoppe JE (1997) Treatment of oropharyngeal candidiasis in immunocompetent infants: a randomised multicentre study of miconazole gel vs nystatin suspension. *Paediatr Infect Dis* 16:288–93.

Jackson DC, Watson JK (2014) Interventions for treating painful nipples among breastfeeding women. *Cochrane Database of Systematic Reviews* (12): CD007366.

Jones W (2018) *Breastfeeding and Medication*, 2nd ed. Routledge.

Kent JC, Ashton E, Hardwick CM, Rowan MK, Chia ES, Fairclough KA, Menon LL, Scott C, Mather-McCaw G, Navarro K, Geddes DT (2015) Nipple pain in breastfeeding mothers: incidence, causes and treatments. *Int J Environ Res Public Health* 12(10):12247–63.

Kirigin Bilos L (2017) Polycystic ovarian syndrome and low milk supply: is insulin resistance the missing link? *Endocr Oncol Metab* 3:49–55.

Morton J, Hall JY, Wong RJ, Thairu L, Benitz WE, Rhine WD (2009) Combining hand techniques with electric pumping increases milk production in mothers of preterm infants. *J Perinatol* 29:757–64.

Neifert MR, Seacat JM, Jobe WE (1985) Lactation failure due to insufficient glandular development of the breast. *Pediatrics* 76(5):823–8.

Nommsen-Rivers LA (2016) Does insulin explain the relation between maternal obesity and poor lactation outcomes? An overview of the literature. *Adv Nutr* 7(2): 407–14.

Smith LJ (2007) Impact of birthing practices on the breastfeeding dyad. *J Midwif Women's Health* 52(6),

Stuebe AM, Meltzer-Brody S, Pearson B, Pedersen C, Grewen K (2015) Maternal neuroendocrine serum levels in exclusively breastfeeding mothers. *Breastfeed Med* 10(4):197–202.

Thomsen AC, Espersen T, Maigaard S (1984) Course and treatment of milk stasis, non-infectious inflammation of the breast and infectious mastitis. *Am J Obstet Gynecol* 149(5):492–5.

van Veldhuizen-Staas CGA (2007) Overabundant milk supply: an alternative way to intervene by full drainage and block feeding. *Int Breastfeed J* 2:11.

WHO (2000) Mastitis causes and management. www.who.int/maternal_child_adolescent/documents/fch_cah_00_13/en/

Woolridge M, Fisher C (1988) Colic, 'overfeeding' and symptoms of lactose malabsorption in the breast-fed baby: a possible artifact of feed management? *Lancet* 2(8607):382–4.

8 Pharmacokinetics of drug transfer into breastmilk

Wendy Jones

Very few drugs are licensed for use by breastfeeding mothers. This does not, in itself, imply risk. Many drugs are prescribed outside of their licence application based on experience. However, there are expert sources which provide information on studies and pharmacokinetics which allow clinicians to make an assessment of the amount of drug passing through milk to the baby and any potential risks. That the manufacturer does not recommend the drug is used should not deter professionals from prescribing after consulting expert sources.

When we prescribe for a breastfeeding mother there are several factors which we need to bear in mind:

- Does the mother's clinical condition need medication?
- How old is the baby and how often is it breastfeeding?
- What information is available from specialist sources – LactMed, Hale and Rowe (2017), Jones (2018)? We can almost invariably expect the *British National Formulary* (BNF) to say that manufacturers advise avoidance. We should not expect the mother to stop breastfeeding unless there is no other alternative medication.
- Is the risk of the drug to the breastfeeding baby low and acceptable to the mother after an informed discussion of the data?

The difficulty is that we are exposing two individuals to the drug – the mother and the baby. However, in many cases the amount passing through milk to the baby is limited. There are several membranes and organs between the mother taking the drug and the baby suckling the milk in which it is contained.

Passage of drugs into breastmilk

The passage of drugs into breastmilk is governed by several factors:

- the oral bioavailability of a drug;
- the half-life of the drug;
- the plasma protein binding;
- the milk–plasma ratio;
- the extent to which the drug undergoes first-pass metabolism;
- the relative infant dose.

We also need to consider the stage of the lactation. Drugs pass freely into breastmilk in the first few days after the birth when the intercellular gaps are wide open to facilitate the passage of immunoglobulins to protect the baby.

The maturity of the baby is also important. A newborn baby has incomplete hepatic and renal function so may not be able to metabolise drugs as readily as an older child. This can lead to extended half-life with some medications, e.g. fluconazole and pethidine. An older baby feeding once or twice a day is also at much less of a risk from the passage of drugs than an exclusively breastfed baby.

When a drug is taken throughout pregnancy the metabolism of the drug is undertaken by the mother. Once the baby is born it has to metabolise anything which it absorbs on its own.

Passage in the immediate postnatal period

Research has shown that more drugs are prescribed for breastfeeding mothers in the immediate postpartum period than at any other time. We prescribe analgesics, laxatives and low-molecular-weight heparinoids without concern because this is a familiar situation on the maternity ward. However, at this time drugs are able to pass freely through the intercellular gaps and reach higher levels in the baby than at any other time during lactation (Figures 8.1–8.3). However, the absolute volume of colostrum is low and hence the level of the drug lower than when lactation is fully established.

Little research has been conducted on the effect of medication passing through milk to the preterm baby. However, babies who are born prematurely are at a greater

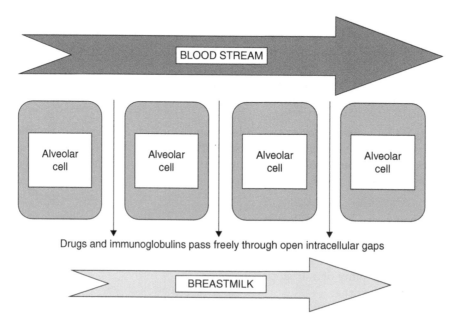

Figure 8.1 Passage of drugs into breastmilk in the first few days after delivery when intercellular junctions remain open

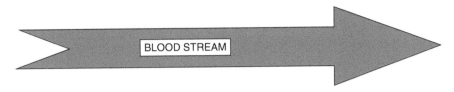

Drugs cannot pass through closed gaps but have to cross cellular membranes

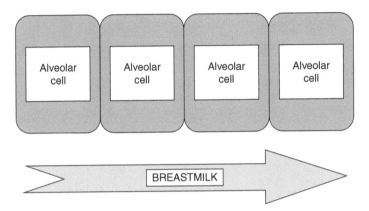

Figure 8.2 Passage of drugs into breastmilk when intercellular junctions have closed 4–10 days after birth. Later in lactation, drugs have to pass across the cell membrane and through the body of the cell or may pass by active transport, e.g. iodine and hence concentrate in breastmilk

risk of necrotising enterocolitis (Herrmann and Carroll 2014) so a decision needs to be made with mothers who need medication chronically that is not compatible with normal breastfeeding or expressing. If such medication is contraindicated, milk banks will do their best to supply donor breastmilk.

Transfer of drugs into breastmilk depends on pharmacokinetics

The oral bioavailability of the drug

This is influenced by the size of the molecule, e.g. insulin (molecular weight > 6,000), low-molecular-weight heparinoids (molecular weights 6,000–20,000), which have to be given by injection as they cannot by absorbed from the gut. The bioavailability is defined as the fraction of the dose which reaches the systemic circulation intact. It is also influenced by first-pass metabolism, where drugs are efficiently cleared by the liver leaving less to reach the systemic circulation. The liver may produce active metabolites which have therapeutic effects of their own, e.g. 6-mercaptopurine. Any drug which has to be given by injection because there is no oral formulation would be compatible with breastfeeding, e.g. gentamicin. The lower the oral bioavailability, the safer the drug is for a breastfeeding mother to take.

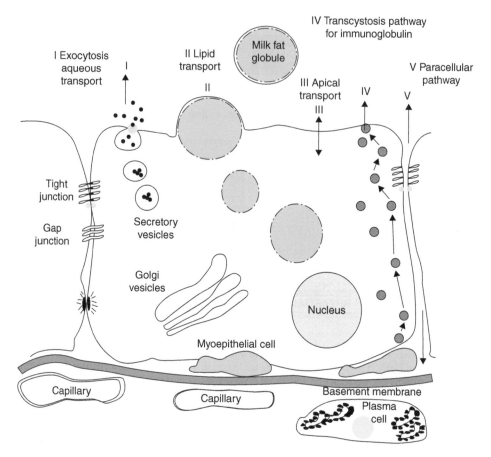

Figure 8.3 Transport of drug molecules across the cell membranes

The influence of the plasma protein binding of the drug

The extent to which a drug is bound to plasma proteins in the maternal bloodstream influences the amount that is available to pass into milk. The more highly bound the drug is, the less that is free to pass through milk to the baby and these drugs are preferred for use in lactation. For example, ibuprofen is more than 99% plasma protein-bound, reflected in the safety during breastfeeding. In the early puerperium drugs that replace bilirubin can cause kernicterus and brain damage, e.g. co-trimoxazole.

The influence of the milk–plasma ratio

This measurement refers to the concentration of the protein-free fractions in milk and plasma. Any ratio over 1 implies that the drug may be unsuitable to be prescribed for a lactating mother. For example, sertraline has a milk–plasma ratio of 0.89, whilst cannabis has ratio of 8, suggesting it concentrates in milk. Likewise, the milk–plasma ratio of iodine is up to 26, which is why it should be avoided during breastfeeding

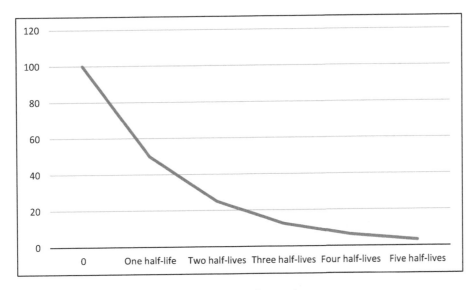

Figure 8.4 Percentage of drug left where half-life is 24 hours

even in dressings. This ratio is not available in standard texts such as the BNF but may be found in specialist texts (Hale 2019).

The influence of the half-life of the drug

The half-life of a drug defines how long it takes to reach steady state and also how long it takes for it to be totally cleared from the mother's body and milk (Figure 8.4). Five half-lives are taken as the closest measure in both cases.

If the half-life of the drug is more than 24 hours the level may begin to accumulate in the baby's body and be more likely to produce adverse effects, e.g. diazepam's half-life 43 hours (Figures 8.5 and 8.6). Drugs with short half-lives are preferred during breastfeeding. In general long-acting/slow-release formulations are better avoided if possible.

The importance of the relative infant dose (RID)

The RID is being increasingly recognised as a valuable guide to the compatibility of a drug taken by a breastfeeding woman. Percentages less than 10% are assumed to be compatible with breastfeeding.

In order to calculate this, the dose in the infant measured in milligrams per kilogram per day is divided by the dose in the mother, also in milligrams per kilogram per day, both doses being derived from studies (Hale 2019):

$$\text{RID} = \frac{\text{dose in the infant (milligrams per kilogramme per day)}}{\text{dose in the mother (milligrams per kilogramme per day)}}$$

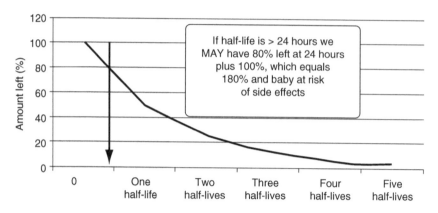

Figure 8.5 Percentage of drug left when half-life exceeds 24 hours

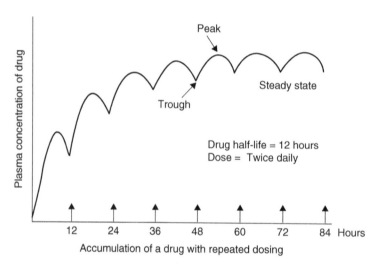

Figure 8.6 Influence of half-life on the accumulation of the drug to steady state. Similarly, the time to reach steady state is governed by the half-life and timing of feeds is only effective before this time to limit medication levels

Licensed for children

Any drug which has a paediatric licence will be compatible for a breastfeeding mother to take and continue to feed as normal. Almost invariably the levels in breastmilk will be subtherapeutic (Figure 8.7). Such drugs are always a compatible option, e.g. antibiotics, mebendazole, antihistamines (ideally non-sedating).

Why are we concerned about prescribing during lactation?

• The information within the BNF is currently in line with manufacturers' rec-ommendation. For example, the entry for sertraline states that it is 'Not known

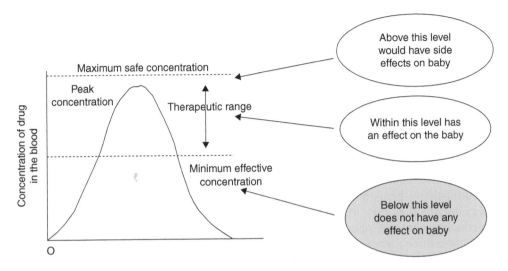

Figure 8.7 Therapeutic levels – overdose to subclinical

to be harmful but consider discontinuing breast-feeding'. When we look at specialist databases, we get a very different view of the compatibility, i.e. that virtually no sertraline gets into breastmilk, so why would we consider discontinuing breastfeeding?

- Licensing: prescribers frequently use medications outside of their product licence. The lack of qualitative or quantitative information within the BNF makes assessment of risk difficult in the face of computer programs reminding us that this drug should not be prescribed during lactation. We are all aware of living in a litigious world with high personal indemnity insurance making us risk-averse.
- Teratogenic drugs: we are all aware of the dangers of taking thalidomide during pregnancy, although it was believed to be compatible from clinical trials. Prescribing these drugs during pregnancy should therefore be avoided. The words pregnancy and lactation are frequently used together. However, the compatibility with respect to the baby is different. In pregnancy drugs can be teratogenic and the Medicines and Healthcare products Regulatory Agency (MHRA) (2019) has provided a guide for contraceptives to be used by mothers taking a teratogenic drug. Teratogenic drugs include angiotensin-converting enzyme (ACE) inhibitors, isotretinoin, lithium, methotrexate and antiepilepsy drugs, particularly valproate and carbimazole. Drugs taken during lactation usually produce short-term effects such as drowsiness, diarrhoea and irritability which cease when the drug is stopped. Anderson et al. (2003) looked at research on all drugs used in lactation where an adverse event had been reported. He found 100 case reports, of which 47 were probably linked and 53 possibly linked.

None of the adverse effects were definitely linked with the amount of drug passing to the baby through milk. Drugs affecting the central nervous system accounted for half of all of the reported events, including all three fatalities – although there were additional factors in all of the latter. In the case of the fatalities one was a baby whose mother used methadone but at the postmortem signs of neglect were identified and abnormalities of the baby's organs; a second was overlaid by her mother who had taken phenobarbital to control epilepsy; and the third was a baby who had already had a near-miss sudden infant death syndrome reaction and whose mother was prescribed a benzodiazepine which could have caused the baby to stop breathing. Sixty-three per cent of the reactions were in neonates and only 4% in babies older than 6 months of age. The limited number of reports is in stark contrast to the perceived risks of prescribing in lactation.

Since Anderson's study we have become aware of the fatality of a baby whose mother was prescribed codeine after delivery (Koren et al. 2006). The baby was born healthy at term after a vaginal delivery. His mother took co-codamol 30/500 for episiotomy pain for 2 weeks. On day 7 the baby became lethargic and had intermittent periods of difficulty in breastfeeding. On day 11 he was taken to a paediatrician because he was described as grey in colour and was breastfeeding poorly. He had regained his birthweight but the following day he was found cyanotic by an ambulance team and despite resuscitation attempts was pronounced dead. At postmortem he was found to have very high levels of morphine in his blood (86 ng/mL compared with an expected level in a neonate exposed to codeine through breastmilk of 2.2 ng/mL). The mother had initially taken two tablets every 6 hours (60 mg four times a day) but had halved the dose when she suffered constipation and somnolence herself. She was subsequently found to have multiple copies of the gene that metabolises codeine into morphine. In adults this has been shown to result in severe opioid toxicity, demonstrated by this mother by her sensitivity to the drug and the side effects she experienced. This geno-type occurs in approximately 1% of people in Finland, Denmark, Greece, Portugal and other Caucasians, but 29% of Ethiopians and 10% of southern Europeans. There are four cases of neonatal apnoea following a dose of 60 mg codeine given to breastfeeding mothers. Although codeine was not detected in the serum of the babies, symptoms resolved when the drug was discontinued (Davis and Bhutani 1985). Other yellow card reports have been submitted to the MHRA.

It is for this reason that we no longer recommend codeine for breastfeeding mothers. However, it is not ethically acceptable to say that the mother cannot have adequate pain relief nor that she should avoid breastfeeding for 15 hours after each dose of codeine. Dihydrocodeine, which has a cleaner metabolism, can be prescribed (see Chapter 9, section on analgesics).

The impact on a mother of being told to stop breastfeeding

Lucy Graney, mother (Figure 8.8), blogs as Little Lifts and the following is an extract from her blog (www.facebook.com/littleliftsblog/).

> Recently I have had some difficulties with my eyes and I have been prescribed a long course of steroids at a relatively high dose. The consultant that I saw explained to me the dosage, and length of time I would be taking the medication for and I informed them that I was breastfeeding.
>
> They asked how old baby was and I told them that she was one year. They aud-ibly scoffed saying 'she is quite old now, can you just stop?' I looked them in the eye and said, no. Then they said, 'well can you just give her formula?' again, no, was my response.

By this point they looked confused and exasperated, after all just stopping breastfeeding seemed like the only option to them. The easiest option and the right option, in their opinion. I asked if there were other alternatives available and their response was, no. I informed them that I would not be stopping feeding and I would research the drugs prescribed.

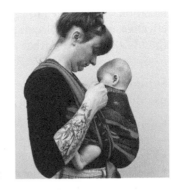

They firmly told me, 'as a medical professional I recommend that you stop breastfeeding and take this medication or your condition will not improve.' They then walked out of the room. This all took place in front of two junior consultants.

Figure 8.8 Lucy Graney

Did they make me feel empowered? No. Did they make me feel like I was being listened to? No. Did they give me options? No. Were they knowledgeable on drugs and breastfeeding? No. Were they wrong? Absolutely.

What I read from expert sources was the total opposite to what I had been advised at the hospital. The drugs at the dose prescribed were in fact safe to take during breastfeeding. The consultant was wrong. To be honest, it was not the fact that they were wrong that bothered me. They were an expert in eyes, not in drugs or breastfeeding, but their attitude was wrong. They made me feel inadequate, dismissed and also frightened.

I agree that the NHS is limited and I do not expect everyone to know everything, but I do think health professionals need the most basic of training in supporting breastfeeding mothers. Even if that just means signposting on to those with more knowledge.

For a professional, it may seem relatively simple to advise a mother that she should stop breastfeeding in order to take a specific medication. The implications vary as to whether this is short-term interruption so that she can 'pump and dump' or long-term so that she needs to wean the baby from the breast.

In both situations the mother needs support and many seek support from voluntary organisations or social media. Despite bottlefeeding being seen as 'the norm' within society, many exclusively breastfed babies do not transfer simply to sucking from a bottle rather than from the breast. The technique is different, the flow rate varies and the taste and temperature vary. In addition, mothers may not own a breast pump or find it easy to pump their milk. It can also be emotionally difficult for a mother to throw her milk down the sink when she knows that it is what her baby needs. Finally, we cannot underestimate the risk of the development of mastitis or subsequent lowering of supply because the breasts have not been drained frequently enough. The baby may in turn become intolerant of the cows' milk protein within formula. What sounds so simple is complex!

Available data on newer medication

It may be tempting to prescribe the most up-to-date medications rather than older ones. The information available on pharmacokinetics and case studies is often slow to be published on new drugs and this may inform our decision making. During lactation we may need to prescribe a drug which is perhaps older but nevertheless still effective, e.g. low-molecular-weight heparinoids rather than novel oral anticoagulants (NOACs), enalapril rather than perindopril.

Summary of points to determine when a drug is likely to be compatible for use during breastfeeding

- if the drug is licensed for paediatric use;
- RID <10%;
- milk–plasma ratio level <1;
- plasma protein binding >90%;
- molecular weight of the drug >200;
- oral bioavailability is poor;
- drug subject to first-pass metabolism;
- no active metabolites;
- studies on use in lactation.

References

Anderson PO, Pochop SL, Manoguerra AS (2003) Adverse drug reactions in breastfed infants: less than imagined. *Clin Pediatr (Phila)* 42(4):325–40.

Davis JM, Bhutani VK (1985) Neonatal apnea and maternal codeine use. *Pediatr Res* 19(4):170A.

Hale TW (2019) *Hale's Medications and Mothers' Milk 2019*. Springer.

Hale TW, Rowe HE (2017) *Medications and Mothers' Milk 2017*. Springer.

Herrmann K, Carroll K (2014) An exclusively human milk diet reduces necrotizing enterocolitis. Breastfeed Med 9(4):184–90.

Jones W (2018) *Breastfeeding and Medication*. Routledge.

Koren G, Cairns J, Chitayat D, Gaedigk A, Leeder SJ (2006) Pharmacogenetics of morphine poisoning in a breastfed neonate of a codeine-prescribed mother. *Lancet* 368(9536):704.

Medicines and Healthcare products Regulatory Agency (MHRA) (2019) Medicines with teratogenic potential: what is effective contraception and how often is pregnancy testing needed? www.gov.uk/drug-safety-update/medicines-with-teratogenic-potential-what-is-effective-contraception-and-how-often-is-pregnancy-testing-needed

9 Compatibility of commonly used drugs in lactation

Wendy Jones

> It is possible to determine the safety of medication according to pharmacokinetics. In this chapter a summary is presented to enable practitioners to determine compatibility of medication with breastfeeding.

Using the pharmacokinetic parameters addressed in Chapter 8, we can look at the drugs most commonly prescribed in general practice to assess their compatibility in lactation. The drugs have been arranged in *British National Formulary* (BNF) categories (NICE 2019a) but due to constraints of space only a summary is provided. Further details can be accessed in Hale and Rowe (2017) and in Jones (2018) as well as via the LactMed database. The pharmacokinetic data have all been taken from Hale. Very few drugs are licensed for use in breastfeeding.

The drugs have been categorised using the following key icons:

- Compatible with breastfeeding   ☺
- Avoid during breastfeeding   ☹
- Use with care during breastfeeding – may be associated with side effects.   ?

Gastrointestinal system

Inflammatory bowel disease (IBD)

There is some evidence of a genetic predisposition to the development of IBD and the use of formula milk particularly in early puerperium, so mothers may be keen to avoid any drug necessitating cessation/interruption of breastfeeding.

Management of acute flare with *prednisolone* dose up to 40 mg a day is compatible with normal breastfeeding. With prolonged high intravenous (IV) doses of hydrocortisone and methylprednisolone, it may be advisable to delay breastfeeding for 4 hours.

Maintenance of remission

- *Azathioprine* – from studies widely used with normal breastfeeding. Relative infant dose (RID) licensed for use in children > 2 years.
- *Mercaptopurine* – metabolite of azathioprine. No studies could be located on this drug alone but, from azathioprine data, levels in milk appear low.

- *Sulfasalazine* – be alert for bloody diarrhoea. RID 0.3–1.1%; licensed for use in children > 2 years.
  - *Mesalazine* – be alert for watery diarrhoea. Negligible amounts in milk. RID 0.12–8.76%.
  - *Balsalazide* – absorbed in colon, not gut, and broken down to mesalazine. No studies located. Be alert for watery diarrhoea.
  - *Olsalazine* – one case study of 1 patient where RID calculated as 0.9%. Monitor for watery diarrhoea.

Monoclonal antibodies

Babies of mothers with IBD on monoclonal antibodies should avoid live vaccines, especially rotavirus due to shedding into faeces. The mother is at risk of contracting virus from these. If vaccination is given, mother should wear gloves and be careful with hand hygiene.

- *Infliximab* – molecular weight 149,100. Poor oral bioavailability, RID 0.32–3.01%.
- *Adalimumab* – molecular weight 148,000. Poor oral bioavailability, RID 0.12%.
- *Golimumab* – molecular weight 150,000. Poor oral bioavailability.
- *Certolizumab pegol* – molecular weight 149,100. Poor oral bioavailability. RID 0.04–0.3%. Licensed for use in breastfeeding.

Laxatives

Laxatives that are compatible with breastfeeding include:

- bulk-forming laxatives;
- osmotic laxatives;
- stool softeners;
- laxative enemas/suppositories;
- stimulant laxatives: bisacodyl, senna, sodium picosulphate;
- bowel-cleansing solutions – normally osmotic laxatives.

Haemorrhoidal preparations

Suppositories and creams are compatible with breastfeeding.

Treatment of anal fissures

- *Glyceryl trinitrate* (GTN) ointment – in one small study all mothers developed headache and/or hot flushes, but no babies reacted.
- *Diltiazem cream* – there are no studies, but oral diltiazem is compatible with breastfeeding, so risk is considered low. GTN is preferred.
- *Botox* – in one study a mother continued to breastfeed after botulinum poisoning with no identified response in the baby. Therapeutic dose of Botox is unlikely to exceed that level.

Antispasmodics

- *Mebeverine* – plasma protein-bound (PPB) 75%, licensed in children. ☺
- *Hyoscine* – PPB 50%, oral bioavailability 81%, licensed in children. ☺
- *Peppermint oil* – undergoes rapid first-pass metabolism, licensed in children. ☺
- *Dicycloverine (dicyclomine)* – used to be used to relieve colic in babies. RID 6.9%. One report of apnoea in a baby exposed through breastmilk (personal communication, N.G. Dahl, Marion Merrell Dow, Inc., 1992, cited in Briggs et al. 2005). Better avoided. ☹
- *Alverine* – one report suggests it is no more effective than placebo (Mitchell et al. 2002). No data on passage into breastmilk. ?

Cardiovascular system

Diuretics ☹

- *Bendroflumethiazide* – in doses of 10 and 15 mg/day it has been used to stop milk supply. There remains a theoretical risk at 2.5 mg, although the amount in milk is not harmful.
- *Furosemide* – no reports of studies in breastmilk but large risk to supply.
- *Indapamide* – assumed also to reduce supply.
- *Spironolactone* – 90% PPB, poor oral bioavailability, RID 2–4.3%. Use only where necessary.

Angiotensin-converting enzyme (ACE) inhibitors

- *Enalapril* – active metabolite enalaprilat, RID 0.07–0.2%. ☺
- *Ramipril* – 56% PPB, oral bioavailability 60%. No studies. ?
- *Lisinopril* – oral bioavailability 25%. No studies. ?
- *Perindopril* – no studies. ?
- *Quinapril* – PPB 97%. One study where active metabolite not identified in milk. ?

Beta-blockers

- *Atenolol* – low PPB, RID 6.6%. If used immediately after birth observe baby for hypoglycaemia. ?
- *Labetolol* – widely used in the perinatal period, 50% PPB, RID 0.2–0.6%. Amount in milk too small to be harmful. ☺
- *Propranolol* – 90% PPB, undergoes first-pass metabolism, RID 0.3–0.5%. Widely used for migraine prophylaxis, in anxiety, with hyperthyroid symptoms. ☺
- *Metoprolol* – milk–plasma (MP) ratio >1 but studies have failed to detect it in breastmilk, undergoes extensive first-pass metabolism, 12% PPB, RID 1.4%. Amount in milk too small to be harmful. ☺
- *Bisoprolol* – oral bioavailability 80%, manufacturer states that <2% in breastmilk, anecdotal reports of use by breastfeeding mothers. ?

Angiotensin II receptor antagonists (sartans)

No evidence of safety from trials. 😞

- *Candestartan* – bioavailability 14%, PPB > 99%.
- *Irbesartan* – oral bioavailability 60–80%, PPB 90%.
- *Losartan* – oral bioavailability 33%, PPB 99.8%.
- *Valsartan* – oral bioavailability 23%, PPB 95%.

Calcium channel blockers

- *Nifedipine* – used to treat Raynaud's phenomenon which can cause painful breastfeeding. Oral bioavailability 50%, PPB 92–98%, RID 2.3–3.4%. Transfers into milk in low levels. 😊
- *Amlodipine* – oral bioavailability 64–90%, PPB 93%, RID 1.72–3.15%. Limited studies showed no adverse effects in breastfed babies. 😊
- *Diltiazem* – oral bioavailability 40–60%, PPB 78%, RID 0.9%. Single case study on mother taking 240 mg/day. 😊
- *Felodipine* – oral bioavailability 20%, PPB >99%, no studies. 😞
- *Lacidipine* – no data. ❓
- *Lercanidipine* – no data. 😞
- *Verapamil* – oral bioavailability 20–35%, PPB 90%, RID 0.22%. Three single-patient studies indicated low levels in breastmilk. 😊

Alpha-blockers

- *Doxazosin* – oral bioavailability 62–69%, PPB 98%, RID 0.58% – 0.87%. Single-patient study indicated low transfer. 😊
- *Prazosin* – oral bioavailability 43–82%, PPB 92–97%, no studies. 😞
- *Terazocin* – no data. ❓

Anticoagulants

- *Warfarin* – oral bioavailability complete, PPB 99%, small and insignificant amounts in breastmilk. 😊
- *Heparin* – molecular weight 12,000–15,000 so cannot transfer into milk or be absorbed by baby. 😊
- *Enoxaprin* – molecular weight 8,000, oral bioavailability zero so cannot transfer into milk or be absorbed by baby. 😊
- *Tinzaparin* – molecular weight <7,500, zero oral bioavailability so cannot transfer into milk or be absorbed by the baby. 😊
- *Dalteparin* – molecular weight 6,000, zero oral bioavailability so cannot transfer into milk or be absorbed by the baby. 😊
- *Fondaparinux* – oral bioavailability 0, PPB 94%, molecular weight 1,728. Unlikely to be passed through breastmilk but no studies. 😊
- *Rivaroxaban* – oral bioavailability 66–100%, PPB 92–95%, RID 1.34. Single case study but baby was not breastfed so no outcome data. 😞

- *Dabigatran* – oral bioavailability 6.5%, PPB 'low'. No studies but transfer expected to be significant. ☹
- *Apixaban* – oral bioavailability 50%, PPB 87%, no studies. ☹

Antiplatelet agents

- *Aspirin* 75–150 mg, oral bioavailability 50–75%, PPB 88–93%, RID 2.5–10.8%. No documented risk association with Reye syndrome. Virtually all metabolised 2–3 hours after dose. ☺
- *Clopidogrel* – oral bioavailability 50%, PPB 98%, metabolite has half-life of 11 days, irreversible inhibition of platelet aggregation may be harmful to baby. No studies. ⊘

Lipid regulation

There is no research on the use of statins during breastfeeding. Cholesterol is important to the development of the baby and the long-term effects of lowered levels are unknown.

- *Simvastatin* – oral bioavailability 5%, PPB 95%, no studies. ☹
- *Atorvastatin* – oral bioavailability 14%, PPB >98%, no studies. ⊘
- *Pravastatin* – oral bioavailability 17%, PPB 50%, no studies. ⊘
- *Rosuvastatin* – oral bioavailability 20%, PPB 88%, RID 0.6–0.77%. Study of one patient but baby was not breastfed so no outcome data. ⊘

Respiratory system

Asthma

- *Beta-adrenoreceptor agonists* – act locally in lungs and limited transfer into blood, let alone milk:
  - *Salbutamol, bambuterol, formoterol, salmeterol, salbutamol, terbutaline.* ☺
- *Corticosteroids*:
  - *Prednisolone* – limited transfer at 40 mg/day, higher doses short term. ☺
- *Inhaled corticosteroids* – act locally in lungs and limited transfer into blood, let alone milk:
  - *Beclometasone, budesonide, fluticasone, mometasone.* ☺
- *Theophylline/aminophylline* – prolonged half-life in neonates, MP ratio 0.67, PPB 56%, oral bioavailability 76%, RID 5.9%. One reported case of irritability. Avoid if possible, especially in young babies. ⊘
- *Leukotriene receptor antagonists*:
  - *Montelukast* – PPB 99%, oral bioavailability 64%, RID 0.68%. Used in children. ☺
  - *Zafirlukast* – PPB >99%, oral bioavailability poor, RID 0.7%. Absorption slowed with food. Used in children > 12 years. ☺

Antihistamines

Antihistamines are widely used by breastfeeding mothers to relieve the symptoms of hayfever. They may also be needed for acute reactions. The latter react more rapidly to the original antihistamines, particularly chlorpheniramine, which may be the better choice for short-term use. Long-term they can cause drowsiness in the baby and reduction in milk supply so should not be used for hayfever.

- Sedating antihistamines
  - *Chlorpheniramine* – PPB 70%, oral bioavailability 25–45%, no studies. Used widely in children. Long-term may cause drowsiness in baby and lowered milk supply. Use for acute allergic reactions. (?)
  - *Promethazine* – PPB 76–93%, oral bioavailability 25%, half-life 16 hours, no studies. Used extensively for hyperemesis and sometimes recommended for insomnia. Long-term may cause drowsiness in baby and lowered milk supply. Use for acute allergic reactions. Due to long half-life may accumulate. (?)
- Non-sedating antihistamines
  - *Loratadine* – PPB 97%, oral bioavailability complete, RID 0.77–1.19%, used in children. (☺)
  - *Cetirizine* – PPB 93%, oral bioavailability 70%, used in children. (☺)
  - *Levocetirizine* – PPB 92%, oral bioavailability complete, no studies but as isomer of cetirizine believed compatible, used in children. (☺)
  - *Desloratadine* – PPB 87%, oral bioavailability good, RID 0.03%, used in children. (☺)
  - *Fexofenadine* – PPB 60–70%, oral bioavailability complete, RID 0.5–0.7%, used in children > 12 years. (☺)
  - *Mizolastine* – no studies, potential to prolong QT interval, long duration of action. Avoid if possible. (?)
- Mucolytics are rarely used except in patients with cystic fibrosis or chronic obstructive airway disease but appear in some cough mixtures, particularly in Ireland, and are included here for completeness. (☺)
  - *Carbocisteine* – no data on levels in breastmilk but used in children.
- Cough preparations – there is little evidence of benefit for the use of cough medicines, but they are still widely used by patients, including breastfeeding mothers, to relieve symptoms. (☺)
- Nasal decongestants.

There is little evidence of benefits of oral decongestants over topical sprays and drops. Steam inhalation and saline douches can be used.

Oral decongestants, particularly pseudoephedrine, have been shown to decrease supply by 24% after a single dose and should be avoided (Aljazaf et al. 2003).

- *Pseudoephedrine* – oral bioavailability 90%, RID 4.7%. The amount passing through milk is not harmful to the baby generally, although irritability has been reported. (☹)
- *Phenylephrine* – oral bioavailability 38%, so unlikely to enter milk in clinically relevant amounts. No studies to show reduction in milk supply but concern exists. (☹)

Topical decongestants: xylometazoline, oxymetazoline are compatible with breastfeeding, as are products such as Olbas Oil, Vick (avoid use close to the baby's face) and First Defence.   ☺

Centrally acting drugs

Hypnotics

Many mothers with anxiety and depression present with symptoms of insomnia. They say that, even when their baby is sleeping soundly, they cannot fall asleep or wake frequently. The use of hypnotics is problematic as the drugs will almost inevitably cross the blood–brain barrier and cause drowsiness in the infant. It is preferable to treat the cause of the insomnia and to refer for cognitive behavioural therapy. N.B.: The drug halves with every half-life that passes but remains in the system for five half-lives. If a mother does not breastfeed overnight following the use of a hypnotic, her supply will begin to diminish but in the short term she risks engorgement and mastitis.

- *Nitrazepam* – PPB 96%, oral bioavailability 90%, half-life 30 hours, RID 2.9%. In a study of nine women no adverse effects were noted in the babies (Matheson et al. 1990a).   (?)
- *Temazepam* – PPB 96%, oral bioavailability 70%, half-life 8–15 hours. In a study of ten mothers (Lebedevs et al. 1992), levels were undetectable in nine babies and no adverse effects were noted.   (?)
- *Zolpidem* – PPB 93%, oral bioavailability 70%, half-life 2.5–5 hours, undergoes extensive first-pass metabolism, RID 0.02–0.18%. One personal communication (Hale 1999) of combination of sertraline and zolpidem resulted in a sedated baby with poor feeding, which resolved on withdrawal of hypnotic.   (?)
- *Zopiclone* – PPB 45%, oral bioavailability 75%, half-life 4–5 hours, RID 1.5%. Matheson et al. (1990b) studied 12 babies whose mothers were given 7.5 mg zopiclone in the early postnatal period. None showed any adverse effects but they were not allowed to breastfeed for 10 hours.   (?)

Anxiolytics

- *Diazepam* – PPB 99%, oral bioavailability complete, RID 7.1, half-life 43 hours. Single doses or short-term, low-dose use for muscle spasm does not seem to present problems but observe for sedation and poor feeding.   (?)
- *Lorazepam* – PPB 85%, oral bioavailability 90%, RID 2.5%, half-life 12 hours. Observe for sedation and poor feeding.   (?)
- *Alprazolam* – PPB 80%, oral bioavailability 90%, RID 8.5%, half-life 12–15 hours.   (?)

Epilepsy

- *Lamotrigine* – PPB 55%. Relatively high plasma levels have been reported in breastfed babies. Neonates are particularly susceptible due to their inability to metabolise the drug if the dosage is not reduced to the pre-pregnancy dosage in the immediate postpartum period. RID is quoted as 9.2–18.3%. Page-Sharp et al.

(2006) studied six breastfeeding women taking a mean dose of 400 mg/day of lamotrigine. Five of the babies were exclusively breastfed and the remaining one fed with half breastmilk and half artificial milk feeds. They determined a RID of 7.6%. No adverse events were noted in any of the infants. In general, infants should be monitored for sedation, feeding difficulties, adequate weight gain and developmental milestones.   (?)

- *Levetiracetam* – Kramer et al. (2002) studied one baby born at 36 weeks and unstable at birth. Following maternal intake of levetiracetam on day seven the baby became hypotonic and fed poorly. The mother was taking multiple medications to control her epilepsy, any of which may have caused the symptoms. Johannessen et al. (2005) studied eight women with maternal doses of levetiracetam up to 3.5 g daily, which produced low levels in milk and no adverse effects in their breastfed infants. The babies of mothers taking levetiracetam should be monitored for drowsiness and adequate weight gain, particularly if the mother is receiving a multiple drug therapy regimen.   (?)

- *Phenytoin* – extensively PPB (90%) but may be displaced by other agents. Rapidly converted to inactive metabolites.   (?)

- *Sodium valproate* – low levels are found in breastmilk but theoretically it is recommended that the baby should be monitored for jaundice and liver damage. Use in lactation less common because it is no longer recommended in pregnancy. Children exposed in utero to valproate are at a high risk of serious developmental disorders (in up to 30–40% of cases) and/or congenital malformations (in approximately 10% of cases) (Medicines and Healthcare products Regulatory Agency (MHRA) 2017).   (?)

- *Carbamazepine* – 75% bound to plasma proteins and has active metabolites. It reaches measurably detectable levels in infant serum but below the therapeutic range. The infant should be monitored for jaundice, drowsiness and adequate weight gain as sedation, poor sucking and hepatic dysfunction have been reported, although rarely.   (?)

- *Topiramate* – only 9–17% protein-bound, and metabolism may be affected by other enzyme-inducing drugs, including other antiepileptic agents. It has been linked to cleft lip with or without cleft palate following first-trimester use (Margulis et al. 2012). Öhman et al. (2002) observed five babies at delivery and followed three of them through lactation. Two to three weeks after delivery two of the breastfed infants had detectable but unquantifiable levels of topiramate and one had an undetectable concentration; MP ratios of around 0.86 were determined and no adverse events were noted.   (?)

- *Phenobarbital* – long half-life can lead to accumulation in baby and sedation. Not advised during lactation.   ☹

Attention deficit disorder

- *Methylphenidate* – PPB 10–33%, oral bioavailability 95%, RID 0.2–0.4%. Studies published on only four mothers, but no adverse effects noted in infants.   (?)

- *Dexamphetamine* – PPB 16–20%, oral bioavailability complete, RID 2.46–7.25%. Observe baby for agitation, insomnia, restlessness, poor feeding.   (?)

- *Lisdexamphetamine* – PPB 16–20%, oral bioavailability 96%, RID 1.8–6.2%. Lisdexamphetamine is rapidly metabolised to dexamphetamine.   (?)

Bipolar disorder

- *Olanzapine* – MP ratio 0.38 and RID 0.28–2.24. From published data, doses up to 20 mg daily produce low levels in milk and undetectable levels in the serum of breastfed infants. Monitor the baby for drowsiness and effective feeding. ⓪

- *Quetiapine* – MP ratio of 0.29, 0.02% – 0.1%. From published data doses of up to 400 mg daily produce low levels in milk. Monitor the baby for drowsiness and effective feeding. ⓪

- *Risperidone* – MP ratio 0.42, limited published information indicates that doses of up to 6 mg daily produce low levels in milk and no observed adverse effects in the babies. Monitor the baby for drowsiness and effective feeding. ⓪

- *Ariprazole* – 87% orally bioavailable and 99% PPB. However, it seems to inhibit prolactin and is associated with a poor milk supply (Mendhekar et al. 2006; Nordeng et al. 2014). ⓪

- *Clozapine* – appears to be distributed into breastmilk in relatively high concentrations. There is one published report of a baby experiencing drowsiness and one who developed agranulocytosis, possibly due to the drug exposure. It should be used with extreme care, if at all (Dev and Krupp 1995). ☹

Depression

Depression in the first year after birth is common and may well be something you see in a routine consultation. If a mother has already had a drug in the past that worked, that may be the best option to prescribe as she already has faith in it and just needs reassurance about use in breastfeeding. To stop breastfeeding is rarely, if ever, necessary unless that is the mother's stated wish. There is a toolkit prepared by the Royal College of General Practitioners (RCGP) (www.rcgp.org.uk/clinical-and-research/resources/toolkits/mental-health-toolkit.aspx).

Selective serotonin re-uptake inhibitors (SSRIs) ☺

- *Sertraline* – PPB 98%, oral bioavailability complete, RID 0.4–2.2%.
- *Citalopram* – PPB 80%, oral bioavailability 80%, RID 3.56–5.37%.
- *Escitalopram* – isomer of citalopram, PPB 56%, oral bioavailability 80%, RID 5.2–7.9%.
- *Fluoxetine* – PPB 94.5%, oral bioavailability complete, RID 1.6–14.6%.
- *Paroxetine* – PPB 95%, oral bioavailability complete, RID 1.2–2.8%.

Tricyclic antidepressants (caution with co-sleeping if they make the mother drowsy)

- *Amitriptyline* – PPB 94.8%, oral bioavailability complete, undergoes first-pass metabolism, RID 1.08–2.8%. ☺
- *Lofepramine* – BNF states: 'The amount secreted into breast milk is too small to be harmful'. ☺
- *Nortriptyline* – PPB 92%, oral bioavailability 51%, RID 1.7–3.36%. ☺
- *Imipramine* – PPB 90%, oral bioavailability 90%, RID 0.1–4.4%. ☺
- *Clomipramine* – PPB 96%, oral bioavailability complete, RID 2.8%. ☺

- *Dosulepin/dothiepin* – oral bioavailability 30%, undergoes extensive first-pass metabolism, RID 0.8–2.2%. ☺
- *Doxepin* – two cases of adverse effects, possibly due to accumulation of metabolite in newborn. Avoid, particularly in neonates. ☹

Serotonin and noradrenaline re-uptake inhibitors

- *Venlafaxine* – PPB 27%, oral bioavailability 45%, RID 6.8–8.1%. Withdrawal after delivery if taken in pregnancy likely. Observe for jitteriness, respiratory distress, cyanosis, apnoea, seizures, temperature instability which may represent discontinuation syndrome. ?
- *Duloxetine* – PPB >90%, oral bioavailability >70%, RID 0.1–1.1%, although studies limited in number. ☺

Alpha$_2$-adrenoreceptor antagonists ☺

- *Mirtazapine* – PPB 85%, oral bioavailability 50%, RID 1.6–6.3%. Studies in doses up to 45 mg but limited in number. No adverse effects noted.

Drugs to treat obesity

- *Orlistat* – PPB >99%, oral bioavailability minimal. Unlikely to enter breastmilk but no studies. Concerns due to high fat content of breastmilk. ?

Labyrinthitis/vertigo

- *Betahistine* – PPB <5%, oral bioavailability complete, but no studies. ?
- *Cinnarazine* – PPB 91%, no studies but licensed for use in children, including for prevention of travel sickness. ☺
- *Prochlorperazine* – PPB 90%, oral bioavailability 12.5%, no studies but anecdotally widely used. BNF states: 'sometimes used in breast-feeding women for short-term treatment of nausea and vomiting'. ☺

Nausea and vomiting

- *Domperidone* – PPB 93%, oral bioavailability 13–17%, RID 0.01–0.35%. May increase milk supply by stimulating prolactin. Use with caution if mother or baby has heart problems or taking any other drugs which may prolong QT interval. ☺
- *Metoclopramide* – PPB 30%, oral bioavailability 30–100%, RID 4.7–14.3%. May increase milk supply by stimulating prolactin. ☺
- *Cyclizine* – no studies but licensed for use in children, including to prevent travel sickness.
- *Ondansetron* – PPB 70–76%, oral bioavailability 60%. No studies but used after caesarean sections and in children (*British National Formulary for Children* (BNFC); NICE 2019b). ☺
- *Hyoscine* – PPB 50%, oral bioavailability 81%, licensed in children. ☺

Analgesics

Paracetamol and non-steroidal anti-inflammatory drugs (NSAIDs) form the mainstay of analgesia.

- *Paracetamol* – PPB 10–25%, oral bioavailability >85%, RID 6.41–24.23%. If an overdose has been taken breastfeeding cannot recommence until blood levels in the mother return to normal. *N*-acetylcysteine levels are low because of poor oral bioavailability (10–30%). Half-life 5–6 hours. ☺
- *Ibuprofen* – PPB > 99%, oral bioavailability 80%, RID 0.12–0.66%. ☺
- *Diclofenac* – PPB 99.7%, oral bioavailability complete. Levels in studies below level of detection. ☺
- *Naproxen* – PPB 99.7%, oral bioavailability 74–99%, RID 3.3%. Despite longer half-life can be used. Three case reports of adverse events in newborns exposed through milk: prolonged bleeding, drowsiness, vomiting. Widely used post-caesarean section after concerns of cardiac risk of diclofenac reduced use. ☺
- *Ketoprofen* – PPB >99%, oral bioavailability 90%, RID 0.3%. ☺
- *Mefenamic acid* – no studies but BNF states: 'amount in milk too small to be harmful'. ☺
- *Celecoxib* – PPB 97%, oral bioavailability 99%, RID 0.3–0.7%. Preferred drug in this class. ☺
- *Meloxicam* – PPB 99.4%, oral bioavailability 89%, but no studies. ⊙?
- *Indometacin* – PPB >90%, oral bioavailability 90%, RID 1.2%. One case of seizure reported in neonate exposed through milk. Avoid. ☹
- *Etoricoxib* – no data.

Opiates

Guidance on opiate prescribing:

> Dihydrocodeine or tramadol can be considered during breastfeeding. This should be at the lowest effective dose and for the shortest duration. Regular use of any opioid in a breastfeeding mother beyond 3 days should be under close medical supervision.
>
> Until more evidence becomes available, consideration should be given to the potential for ultra rapid metabolism with dihydrocodeine or tramadol use. If significant opioid adverse effects develop in the mother, this could suggest the possibility that she is an ultra rapid metaboliser and that the risk of adverse effects in the infant may be increased. All breastfeeding mothers should be informed of the potential problems and advised to withhold breastfeeding if symptoms develop and seek medical advice.
>
> Infants exposed to either dihdrocodeine or tramadol should be monitored for sedation, breathing difficulties, constipation, difficulty feeding and adequate weight gain.
>
> If adverse effects develop in breastfeeding infants, the opioid should preferably be replaced by an alternative non-opioid analgesic.
>
> (Specialist Pharmacy Services 2018)

- *Codeine* – PPB 7%, oral bioavailability complete, RID 0.6–8.1%. Some mothers concentrate the morphine metabolites of codeine into milk and there has been at least one fatality (Koren et al. 2006). Despite being the mainstay of analgesia for many years, codeine is no longer recommended for breastfeeding mothers (European Medicines Agency 2013; MHRA 2013a).   (?)
- *Dihydrocodeine* – cleaner metabolism than codeine, oral bioavailability approximately 20%, subject to first-pass metabolism. Opiate of choice in breastfeeding women.   (☺)
- *Oxycodone* – PPB 45%, oral bioavailability 60–87%, RID 1.01–8%. Multiple case reports of causing drowsiness in breastfed babies exposed through their mother's milk together with breathing and feeding difficulties. Marked drowsiness reported at doses over 30 mg/day.   (?)
- *Tramadol* – PPB 20%, oral bioavailability 60%, RID 2.86%. Observe for sedation and poor feeding. Has an active metabolite. Study of 75 mothers who were given 100 mg every 6 hours after caesarean birth showed no adverse events.   (?)
- *Aspirin* – should not be used at analgesic dose routinely, compatible with breastfeeding at 75–150 mg/day. If taken accidentally risk of adverse events is low as no reports associating passage through breastmilk and Reye's syndrome have been documented. Avoiding breastfeeding for 2–3 hours eliminates even minor risk.   (?)
- *Morphine* – PPB 35%, oral bioavailability 26%, RID 9.09–35%. Infants under 4 weeks of age have a prolonged elimination half-life and clearance does not approach adult levels until 2 months of age. It is important to be aware of respiratory difficulties with premature babies or others at risk of apnoea. The oral absorption of morphine is very poor and first-pass metabolism is high. It is therefore frequently used post-caesarean section as Oramorph solution.   (?)
- *Pethidine* – PPB 65–80%, oral bioavailability <50%, RID 1.1–13.3%. Pethidine undergoes rapid first-pass clearance by the liver, but it is cleared very much more slowly by infants of less than 3 months because of hepatic immaturity. The active metabolite norpethidine is excreted by the kidneys and may also accumulate in neonates who have inherently low kidney function. The average half-life in young babies is estimated to be 11 hours but can range from 3 to 60 hours. Single dose, e.g. as part of sedative procedure for colonoscopy, does not preclude normal breastfeeding as soon as the mother is awake and alert.   (?)

Muscle spasm

Sometimes analgesia is insufficient to reduce pain, e.g. in acute back pain where there is a spasm of the muscles.

- *Diazepam* – PPB 99%, oral bioavailability complete, RID 0.88–7.14%, half-life 43 hours. Long-term use would lead to accumulation but anecdotal reports of low-dose diazepam over 2–3 days to relieve muscle spasm indicate no adverse effects. Appropriate to use for anxiety before procedure or anxiety over a flight as a single dose.   (?)
- *Methocarbamol* – PPB 46–50%, oral bioavailability complete, but no studies in breastmilk.   (?)

Local inflammation of joints

- Local corticosteroid injection anaesthetics can be used during breastfeeding without interruption. The level of steroid released slowly over time is below the level known to be safe in oral steroids. ☺
- Topical anti-inflammatory creams, gels, ointments and patches can be used without interruption as absorption through the skin will be less than that known to be safe via oral absorption. ☺

Migraine

Triptans

- *Sumatriptan* – PPB 14–21%, oral bioavailability 14%, RID 3.5%. Due to poor bioavailability no need to discard milk for 12 hours as recommended by the manufacturer. ☺
- *Rizatriptan* – PPB 14%, oral bioavailability 45%. No studies. (?)
- *Naratriptan* – PPB 29%, oral bioavailability 74%. No studies. (?)
- *Frovatriptan* – PPB 15%, oral bioavailability, 30%. No studies. (?)
- *Almotriptan* – PPB 35%, oral bioavailability 70%. No studies. (?)
- *Zolmitriptan* – PPB 25%, oral bioavailability 40%. No studies. (?)

Over-the-counter remedies

- *Migraleve Pink* – contain paracetamol, codeine and buclizine – see codeine information above. No data on buclizine but single use unlikely to cause problems for a breastfed baby. (?)
- *Migraleve Yellow* – contain paracetamol and codeine – see codeine information above. (?)

Analgesics plus drugs to alter gastric motility

- *Paracetamol plus metoclopramide* – safety as per individual ingredients. ☺
- *Aspirin plus metoclopramide* – avoid, although risk of single dose is low. ☹

Ergotamine-containing drugs – avoid ☹

Neuropathic pain

- *Amitriptyline* – PPB 94.8%, oral bioavailability complete, RID 1.08–2.8%. Be aware of co-sleeping risk. Amount in milk too small to be harmful. ☺
- *Gabapentin* – PPB <3%, oral bioavailability 50–60%, RID 6.6%. There may be neonatal withdrawal if used in pregnancy. Be aware of co-sleeping risk, observe baby for sedation and poor feeding. (?)
- *Pregabalin* – unbound, oral bioavailability 90%, RID 7.18%. One study of ten mothers and babies but no baby was breastfed. (?)

Smoking cessation

Maternal smoking is one of the highest risks for sudden infant death syndrome (SIDS). Any method of smoking cessation using patches, gum, sprays, tablets and so on will result in a lower level of nicotine passed to the baby. There is some evidence that smoking makes babies more at risk of colic and mothers who smoke, in general, give up breastfeeding sooner than others. Breastfeeding continues to have advantages over formula feeding even if the mother smokes.

- *Varenicline* – PPB <20%, oral bioavailability 90%, half-life 24 hours. No studies. (?)
- *Bupropion* – PPB 84%, oral bioavailability 85%, RID 0.11–1.99%. Two cases of seizures reported and anecdotal reports of reduction in milk supply. (?)

Vaping (electronic cigarettes) (?)

Eissenberg (2010) determined that, relative to a cigarette, ten puffs from electronic nicotine delivery devices (e-cigarettes) with a 16-mg nicotine cartridge delivered little to no nicotine. Based on these findings, it may be concluded that the amount of nicotine that transfers into breastmilk after an acute inhalation of an e-cigarette is probably minimal. However, Etter and Bullen (2011) studied 3,587 smokers using e-cigarettes and reported that an average e-cigarette user inhales up to 120 puffs/day, equivalent to five refills per day. Currently there are few studies on long-term use of electronic devices, let alone exposure of a breastfed infant. As with cigarettes, use of these devices away from the baby would be recommended (Czogola et al. 2014), as nicotine exposure continues, although not the other products released by tobacco.

Illicit substance withdrawal

- *Methadone* – PPB 89%, oral bioavailability 50%, RID 1.9–6.5%. Evidence from studies of safety to 105 mg/day. Abrupt cessation of breastfeeding can lead to neonatal withdrawal. (?)
- *Buprenorphine* – PPB 96%, oral bioavailability 70%, RID 0.09–2.52%. Sublingual doses produce low levels in milk if not below level of detection. (?)

Alcohol

- *Alcohol* – PPB zero, oral bioavailability 100%, RID 16%. Occasional social drinking is compatible with breastfeeding within the NHS-suggested limits of consumption for women. Binge drinking may result in high levels so baby should not be breastfed until 1 hour has passed for every unit drunk. If a mother is drinking alcohol, she should not co-sleep. (?)

Infection

Penicillins (all licensed for paediatric use) ☺

- *Phenoxymethylpenicillin* – trace amounts in breastmilk.

- *Amoxycillin* – RID 1%.
- *Co-amoxiclav* – RID 0.9%.
- *Co-fluampicil* – trace amounts in breastmilk.
- *Flucloxacillin* – trace amounts in breastmilk.

Cephalosporins (all licensed for paediatric use)   ☺

- *Cefaclor* – RID 0.4–0.8%.
- *Cefalexin* – RID 0.39–1.47%.
- *Cefadroxil* – RID 0.8–1.3%.
- *Cefradine* – trace amounts in breastmilk.
- *Cefuroxamine* – RID 0.6–2%.

Tetracyclines (not suitable for long courses, e.g. to treat acne, rosacea)

- *Doxycycline* – PPB 90%, oral bioavailability 90–100%, RID 4.2–13.3%. Not suitable for long courses but courses up to 3 weeks acceptable without risk of damage to teeth and bones as the drug is chelated by the calcium in milk.   ⊘
- *Lymecycline.*   ☹
- *Minocycline.*   ☹
- *Oxytetracycline.*   ☹

Aminoglycosides   ☺

- *Gentamicin* – PPB <10–30%, oral bioavailability <1%, RID 2.1%. Only risk is in neonates where the drug may cross through the open junctions between the cells.
- *Neomycin* – suitable for use in eye and ear drops
- *Vancomycin* – PPB 20–50%, oral bioavailability negligible.
- *Teicoplanin* – licensed for use in children. Not absorbed from the gastrointestinal tract. No studies.

Macrolides   ☺

Observe for pyloric stenosis in neonates but current evidence is that the risk is low (Abdellatif et al. 2019).

- *Erythromycin* – RID 1.4–1.7%. Licensed for paediatric use.
- *Azithromycin* – RID 5.9%. Licensed for paediatric use.
- *Clindamycin* – PPB 94%, oral bioavailability 90%, RID 0.9–1.8%. Licensed for paediatric use. One case of pseudomembranous colitis reported but baby exposed to several antibiotics in rapid succession through breastmilk.
- *Clarithromycin* – RID 2.1%. Licensed for paediatric use.

Other antibiotic agents

- *Trimethoprim* – RID 3.9–9%. Licensed for paediatric use.   ☺
- *Nitrofurantoin* – RID 6.8%. Licensed for paediatric use. Use with care in glucose-6-phosphate dehydrogenase (G6PD)-deficient infants.   ☺

Quinolones

- *Ciprofloxacin* – PPB 40%, oral bioavailability 50–85%, RID 0.44–6.34%. Given directly to young rats, it causes a type of juvenile arthritis but not seen in the amount passing through breastmilk. Use only if no other antibiotic is suitable. Avoid taking with NSAIDs to reduce risk of convulsions. ☺
- *Ofloxacin* – PPB 32%, oral bioavailability 98%, RID 3.1%. Avoid if possible because studies limited. ?
- *Levofloxacin* – enantiomer of ofloxacin, RID 10.5–17.2%. Avoid if possible. ?
- *Moxifloxacin* – no studies. ?
- *Norfloxacin* – no studies. ?
- *Metronidazole* – PPB <20%, oral bioavailability complete, RID 12.6–13.5%. Studies show no untoward effects at a dose of 200–400 mg three times a day. Said to alter taste of milk but anecdotal reports suggest this is masked by maternal garlic consumption. ☺

Antifungals

- *Fluconazole* – PPB 11–12%, oral bioavailability >90%, RID 16.4–21.5%. Licensed for paediatric use. Widely used as a single dose to treat vaginal thrush and for courses up to 2 weeks to treat nipple thrush. ☺
- *Itraconazole* – PPB 99.8%, oral bioavailability 55%, RID 0.2%. Absorption unlikely in the pH of the stomach of a breastfed baby. ☺
- *Terbinafine* – PPB 99%, oral bioavailability 80%. Published studies of only two patients but extensive first-pass metabolism. Topical application compatible with breastfeeding. ☺
- *Nystatin* – oral bioavailability zero and plasma levels undetectable after maternal use. Use in the treatment of oral *Candida* in infants shows poor success and miconazole gel is preferable. ☺

Antivirals

- *Aciclovir* – PPB 9–33%, oral bioavailability 15–30%, RID 1.09–1.53%. Licensed for paediatric use. Application of cream, except to nipples, is compatible with breastfeeding. ☺
- *Famciclovir* – PPB < 20%, oral bioavailability 69–85%, no data from studies. More bioavailable than aciclovir, which would be preferred drug. ?
- *Valaciclovir* – PPB 9–33%, oral bioavailability 54%, RID 4.7%. Rapidly metabolised to aciclovir. ☺
- *Oseltaivir* – PPB 42%, oral bioavailability 75%, RID 0.47%. Licensed for paediatric use and widely used for acute influenza. ☺

Threadworm

- *Mebendazole* – PPB high, oral bioavailability 2–10%, licensed for paediatric use from 6 months. Even if breastfed child needs his/her own dose, breastfeeding can continue as normal as amount in milk is so low. No need to 'pump and dump' milk as recommended by the manufacturer.

Endocrine system

Diabetes

Insulin

The molecular size of insulin means that it cannot be absorbed from breastmilk. One study shows that babies breastfed by mothers using insulin do not alter their blood glucose levels. However, mothers should check their blood sugars regularly as breastfeeding can alter them. In general, lower doses can be used or more calories consumed. Care with risk of hypoglycaemia overnight should be taken with suitable snacks available.

Sulfonylureas

- *Glibenclamide* – no data.
- *Gliclazide* – no data.
- *Glimepiride* – PPB > 99.5%, oral bioavailability 100%, no studies but levels in rat pups elevated.
- *Glipizide* – PPB 98–99%, oral bioavailability 90–100%. In two studies babies breastfed by mothers taking this drug had normal blood glucose and blood levels of drug below the level of detection.
- *Tolbutamide* – PPB 93%, oral bioavailability complete, RID 0.004–0.02%. Studies in two patients showed low levels in breastmilk.

Biguanides

- *Metformin* – PPB minimal, oral bioavailability 50%, RID 0.3–0.7%. Large studies showed low levels in breastmilk and no adverse events in babies. Widely used for polycystic ovary syndrome (PCOS) where it can increase milk supply anecdotally.

Dipeptidylpeptidase-4-inhibitors (gliptins)

- *Alogliptin* – no data.
- *Linagliptin* – PPB 70–80%, oral bioavailability 30%, no studies but does not appear to lower blood sugars in normal subjects.
- *Saxagliptin* – no data.
- *Vildagliptin* – PPB 9.3%, oral bioavailability 85%, no studies but does not appear to lower blood sugars in normal subjects.

Glucagon-like peptide1 receptor agonists (no data)

- *Albiglutide, dulaglutide, exanatide, liraglutide, lixisenatide.*

Meglitinides (no data)   🙁

- *Nateglinide, repaglinide.*

Thioglitazones   🙁

- *Pioglitazone* – no data.

Osteoporosis   🙂

Calcium and vitamin D preparations can be used during breastfeeding. Concern has been expressed about the risk of hypocalcaemia in babies (nausea, vomiting, weight loss, thirst, weight loss) but one of the manufacturers of high-dose vitamin D suggests that this has not been identified in breastfed infants exposed through breastmilk. A supplement of 6,400 units a day is needed before the infant does not need his/her own supplement of 10 μg/day (Hollis and Wagner 2004). The normal level of vitamin D supplementation for the breastfeeding mother is 10 μg (400 units per day). Bone density falls during breastfeeding but returns to higher levels after breastfeeding (www. unicef.org.uk/babyfriendly/news-and-research/baby-friendly-research/maternal-health-research/maternal-health-research-bone-density/).

Bisphosphonates

- *Alendronic acid* – PPB 78%, oral bioavailability <0.7%, no studies but levels in plasma below level of detection.
- *Ibandronic acid* – PPB 85.7–99.5%, oral bioavailability 0.6%. No studies but pharmacokinetics suggest low levels in breastmilk.
- *Pamidronate* – oral bioavailability very low. Study of one patient showed breastmilk levels below limit of detection.
- *Risedronate* – oral bioavailability 0.63% but no studies.
- *Zoledronic acid* – no data.

Thyroid

- *Levothyroxine* – PPB 99%, oral bioavailability 50–80%. Very low levels in breastmilk and not enough to affect thyroid levels of infant through breastmilk. Too low a supplementation level can inhibit lactation and produce low milk supply.   🙂
- *Carbimazole* – PPB zero, oral bioavailability complete, RID 2.3–5.3%. Prodrug of methimazole. Studies up to 40 mg/day show low levels in breastmilk, insufficient to suppress thyroid level in breastfed infant (Johansen et al. 1982). Thyroid suppression is believed to occur only when plasma levels exceed 50–100 ng/mL (Rylance et al. 1987). Caution re use in pregnancy (MHRA 2019).   🙂
- *Propylthiouracil* – PPB 80–95%, oral bioavailability 50–95%, RID 1.8%. Studies show levels in breastmilk too low to produce adverse events.   🙂

Contraception

The progesterone-only pill (POP) is widely used by breastfeeding mothers. Anecdotal reports of reduction in milk supply, particularly if initiated before 6 weeks postpartum, have been seen by many lactation specialists. With this in mind, it is suggested that a 1-month trial of oral POP is recommended before use of depot preparations.

Combined hormonal contraception (CHC) is currently recommended by the most recent UK Medical Eligibility Criteria (UKMEC) guidelines (2016) (www.fsrh.org/ukmec/): 'Based on breastfeeding status alone, CHC can be used by breastfeeding women safely after 6 weeks following childbirth'. This is at variance with the previous guidelines that the combined pill is not suitable for a breastfeeding mother in the first 6 months after delivery and with the experience of many breastfeeding workers and is currently a cause for concern. Decisions should be made with mothers fully informed about the risk of initiating contraception early.

Emergency hormonal contraception (EHC) relies on two products, levonorgestrel and ulipristal. Despite manufacturers' recommendations to 'pump and dump' for 8 hours after levonorgestrel and 7 days after ulipristal, there is no evidence of risk from continuing to breastfeed as normal (www.sps.nhs.uk/articles/emergency-contraception-and-breast-feeding/). The insertion of a coil for delayed access to EHC does not affect breastmilk or supply.

Suppression of lactation

The routine suppression of lactation is not recommended by the use of medication. It may be suggested following a neonatal death, although some mothers have expressed a preference to donate their breastmilk for use by preterm babies via milk banks instead.

- *Bromocriptine* – PPB 90–96%, oral bioavailability < 28%. Hale reports that:

  > In 2015, the French pharmacovigilance program published a review of the adverse events associated with bromocriptine use to cease lactation. This group reported 105 serious adverse reactions including cardiovascular (70.5%), neurological (14.4%) and psychiatric (8.6%) events. There were also two fatalities, one 32-year-old female had a myocardial infarction with an arrhythmia, and a 21-year-old female had an ischemic stroke.

  This drug is banned for suppression of lactation in the USA.

- *Cabergoline* – PPB 40–42%, oral bioavailability complete, no data on levels in breastmilk. May produce cessation of breastmilk supply that mother later regrets.

Enhancement of lactation

Mothers with low milk supply may benefit from the prescription of domperidone and metoclopramide which increase supply through increasing prolactin levels.

The use of domperidone has decreased following concerns by the MHRA (2013b) about the risk of adverse cardiac events. It should not be used where either mother or baby has had cardiac symptoms or is taking another drug which prolongs QT interval. The amount of either drug in breastmilk is low. Domperidone has widely been used to support mothers of preterm infants who are pumping rather than breastfeeding for weeks.

- *Metoclopramide* – PPB 30%, oral bioavailability 30–100%, RID 4.7–14.3%. Has been widely used in the past but can precipitate depression in the mother.   ☺
- *Domperidone* – PPB 93%, oral bioavailability 13–17%, RID 0.01% – 0.35%. Use with caution if mother or baby has heart problems or when taking any other drugs which may prolong QT interval.   ☺
- *Fenugreek* – a herb widely used to increase milk supply but poor evidence of efficacy from studies. Can destabilise blood sugars and produce asthma exacerbation. The transfer of fenugreek into milk is unknown but untoward effects have only rarely been reported. One case of suspected gastrointestinal bleeding in a premature infant has been reported.   ☺

Termination of pregnancy or treatment of incomplete miscarriage

- *Misoprostol* – PPB 80–90%, oral bioavailability complete, RID 0.04%. Has in the past been suggested to avoid breastfeeding for 4 hours but passage is so small that this is probably unnecessary.   ☺
- *Mifepristone* – PPB 99.2%, oral bioavailability 69%. Transfer into milk negligible.   ☺

Treatment of ectopic pregnancy

- *Methotrexate* – PPB 50%, oral bioavailability 20–95%, RID 0.11–0.95%. Contraindicated to treat rheumatoid arthritis on an ongoing basis. However, used as a single dose (50 mg/m²) for ectopic pregnancy. May need to be increased to 4 days for higher doses >75 mg (Hale 2019).   ☺

Topical preparations

Eye drops   ☺

The passage of eye drops into breastmilk is significantly reduced by placing pressure over the tear duct by the corner of the eye for 1 minute or more (Figure 9.1), then removing the excess solution with an absorbent tissue. Chloramphenicol, fusidic acid, gentamicin, neomycin, hydrocortisone, ciprofloxacin, levofloxacin and ofloxacin can all be used safely during lactation.

Ear drops   ☺

The passage of ear drops into breastmilk is low due to limited blood supply from the outer-ear canal. For example, gentamicin, neomycin, ciprofloxacin, levofloxacin,

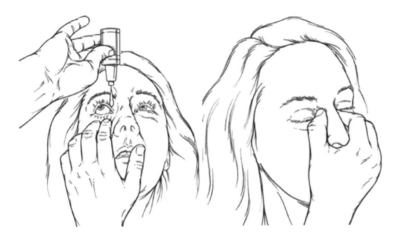

Figure 9.1 Nasolacrimal occlusion
Source: https://www.hopkinsmedicine.org/wilmer/services/glaucoma/book/chapter_how_to_
succeed_with_drops.html

ofloxacin and so on can safely be used during lactation. This includes drops to soften
ear wax.

Nasal drops   😊

Most nasal drops act only locally within the nasal passages and do not pass into
breastmilk, e.g. xylometazoline, steroidal nasal drops and sprays; fluticasone nasules
can be safely used during lactation.

Podiatry surgery   😊

Although many products for podiatry use suggest that they should not be used during
breastfeeding in the patient information leaflet, the absorption through skin will be
low. Treatment of corns, verrucas, cracked heels and ingrowing toenails (involving
local anaesthetic, phenol or sodium hydroxide) can continue as normal without risk
to the baby.

Vaccinations

Vaccinations for hepatitis A and hepatitis B, typhoid, whooping cough, measles,
mumps and rubella (MMR), influenza, meningitis, chickenpox, pneumonia, polio and
BCG can all continue as normal whilst a mother is breastfeeding (www.gov.uk/govern-
ment/collections/immunisation-against-infectious-disease-the-green-book). If a mother
is taking biological agents, the baby should not receive the rotavirus vaccination as the
mother may be infected through viral fragments shed into faeces. If it is chosen to continue with vaccination, she would benefit from using vinyl groups to reduce risk.   😊
There is some evidence of transmission of yellow fever vaccination in babies under
2 months of age. This stems from a case in Brazil in 2009 when a 23-day-old breastfed
infant developed fever and seizures 8 days after the mother received the yellow fever

vaccine. A 5-week-old baby in Canada developed yellow fever encephalitis 30 days after his mother was given the vaccination. It is recommended that immunisation of a mother with a baby under 9 months is avoided if possible.

Anaesthetics

General anaesthetics

There is no evidence that any of the agents used during general anaesthesia justifies any delay in breastfeeding as normal as soon as the mother is awake and alert.

- *Anaesthetics*: propofol, thiopental, etomidate, ketamine, sevoflurane, isoflurane, desflurane.
- *Neuromuscular blockers*: rocuronium, vecuronium, atracurium, suxamethonium, neostigmine, sugammadex.

Local anaesthetics

Local anaesthetics are poorly absorbed even if they pass into milk so after procedures such as dental, sutures and biopsy mothers can breastfeed as normal.

Conscious sedation

Babies can be breastfed as normal as soon as the mother is awake and alert after the procedure.

- *Pethidine* – PPB 65–80%, oral bioavailability <50%, RID 1.1–13.3%. Can be used as a single dose for sedation with normal breastfeeding
- *Fentanyl* – PPB 80–85%, oral bioavailability 50–75%, RID 2.9–5%.
- *Midazolam* – PPB 97%, oral bioavailability 40–50%, RID 0.63%. Previous guidelines that breastfeeding should be avoided for 4 hours in babies under 2 months of age are based on one study where mothers of babies < 6 days old were given 15 mg/day as hypnotics compared to 5 mg nitrazepam. The maximum level of midazolam in breastmilk was 9 µg/L. After 4 hours the level was undetectable (Matheson et al. 1990a).

References

Abdellatif ME, Ghozy S, Kamel MG, Elawady SS Ghorab MME Attia AW, Le Huyen TT, Duy DTV Hirayama K, Huy NT (2019) Association between exposure to macrolides and the development of infantile hypertrophic pyloric stenosis: a systematic review and meta-analysis. *Eur J Pediatr* 178(3):301–14.

Aljazaf K, Hale TW, Ilett KF, Hartmann PE, Mitoulas LR, Kristensen JH, Hackett LP (2003) Pseudoephedrine: effects on milk production in women and estimation of infant exposure via breastmilk. *Br J Clin Pharmacol* 56(1):18–24.

Briggs GG, Freeman RK, Yaffe SJ (2005) *Drugs in Pregnancy and Lactation*, 7th ed. Baltimore: Williams & Wilkins.

Czogola J, Goniewicz M, Fidelus B, Zielinsa-Danch W, Travers M, Sobczak A (2014) Second hand exposure to vapors from electronic cigarettes. *Nicotine Tob Res* 16(6):655–62.

Dev VJ, Krupp P (1995) Adverse event profile and safety of clozapine. *Rev Contemp Pharmacother* 6:197–208.

Eissenberg T (2010) Electronic nicotine delivery devices: ineffective nicotine delivery and craving suppression after acute administration. *Tob Control* 19(1):87–8.

Etter JF, Bullen C (2011) Electronic cigarette: users profile, utilization, satisfaction and perceived efficacy. *Addiction* 106(11):2017–28.

European Medicines Agency (2013) Restrictions on use of codeine for pain relief in children – CMDh endorses PRAC recommendation. Press Release. EMA/385716/2013. 28 June.

Hale TW, Rowe HE (2017) *Medications and Mothers' Milk 2017*. Springer.

Hollis BW, Wagner CL (2004) Vitamin D requirements during lactation: high-dose maternal supplementation as therapy to prevent hypovitaminosis D for both the mother and the nursing infant. *Am J Clin Nutr* 80(Suppl 6):1752S–8S.

Johannessen SI, Helde G, Brodtkorb E (2005) Levetiracetam concentrations in serum and in breast milk at birth and during lactation. *Epilepsia* 46:775–7.

Johansen K, Andersen AN, Kampmann JP, Molholm Hansen JM, Mortensen HB (1982) Excretion of methimazole in human milk. *Eur J Clin Pharmacol* 23(4):339–41.

Jones W (2018) *Breastfeeding and Medication*. Routledge.

Koren G, Cairns J, Chitayat D, Gaedigk A, Leeder SJ (2006) Pharmacogenetics of morphine poisoning in a breastfed neonate of a codeine-prescribed mother. *Lancet* 368(9536):704.

Kramer G, Hosli I, Glanzmann R, Holzgreve W (2002) Levetiracetam accumulation in human breastmilk. *Epilepsia* 43(Suppl. 7):105.

Lebedevs TH, Wojnar-Horton RE, Yapp P, Roberts MJ, Dusci LJ, Hackett LP, Ilett KF (1992) Excretion of temazepam in breast milk. *Br J Clin Pharmacol* 33(2):204–6.

Margulis AV, Mitchell AA, Gilboa SM, Werler MM, Mittleman MA, Glynn RJ, HernandezDiaz S (2012) National Birth Defects Prevention Study. Use of topiramate in pregnancy and risks of oral clefts, *Am J Obstet Gynecol* 207(5):405.e1–7.

Matheson I, Lunde PK, Bredesen JE (1990a) Midazolam and nitrazepam in the maternity ward: milk concentrations and clinical effects. *Br J Clin Pharmacol* 30(6):787–93.

Matheson I, Sande HA, Gaillot J (1990b) The excretion of zopiclone into breast milk. *Br J Clin Pharmacol* 30(2):267–71.

Mendhekar DN, Sunder KR, Andrade C (2006) Aripiprazole use in pregnant schizoaffective woman. *Bipolar Disord* 8:229–300.

MHRA (2013a) Codeine for analgesia: restricted use in children because of reports of morphine toxicity. *Drug Saf Update* 6(12).

MHRA (2013b) Metoclopramide: risk of neurological adverse effects – restricted dose and duration of use (August 2013). www.gov.uk/drug-safety-update/metoclopramide-risk-of-neurological-adverse-effects

MHRA (2017) Valproate and developmental disorders: new alert asking for patient review and further consideration of risk minimisation measures. MHRA.

MHRA (2019) Carbimazole: increased risk of congenital malformations; strengthened advice on contraception. www.gov.uk/drug-safety-update/carbimazole-increased-risk-of-congenital-malformations-strengthened-advice-on-contraception

Mitchell SA, Mee AS, Smith GD, Palmer KR, Chapman RW (2002) Alverine citrate fails to relieve the symptoms of irritable bowel syndrome: results of a double-blind, randomized, placebo-controlled trial, Aliment. *Pharmacol Ther* 16:1187–95.

NICE (2019a) *British National Formulary* (BNF). https://bnf.nice.org.uk

NICE (2019b) *British National Formulary for Children* (BNFC). https://bnfc.nice.org.uk

Nordeng H, Gjerdalen G. Brede WR, Michelsen LS, Spigset O (2014) Transfer of aripiprazole to breast milk: a case report. *J Clin Psychopharmacol* 34(2):272–5.

Öhman I, Vitols S, Luef G, Söderfeldt B, Tomson T (2002) Topiramate kinetics during delivery, lactation, and in the neonate: preliminary observations. *Epilepsia* 43:1157–60.

Page-Sharp M, Kristensen JH, Hackett LP, Beran RG, Rampono J, Hale TW, Kohan R, Ilett KF (2006) Transfer of lamotrigine into breastmilk. *Ann Pharmacother*,40:1470–1, letter.

Rylance GW, Woods CG, Donnelly MC, Oliver JS, Alexander WD (1987) Carbimazole and breastfeeding. *Lancet* 1(8538):928.

Specialist Pharmacy Services (2018) Which weak opioids can be used during breastfeeding? Considering the evidence for codeine, dihydrocodeine, and tramadol. www.sps.nhs.uk/category/medicine/tramadol/

10 Supporting breastfeeding women with mental health issues

Bethany Chapman

Current statistics suggest that up to one in five women report a diagnosable mental health issue within the perinatal period, although this is likely to be underreported, with many more suffering in silence. Some mothers are concerned that their decision to breastfeed may be blamed for their issues and the risks of medication are for them exaggerated by anxiety that they may be told to stop breastfeeding.

Traditionally the focus in primary care has been identifying postnatal depression using DSM 5, with anxiety disorders and birth traumas being widely ignored. However, we are starting to recognise that the perinatal period can trigger or aggravate other mental health disorders too, such as obsessive compulsive disorder, generalised anxiety and low self-esteem issues. Mothers that feel out of control during labour may become distressed, triggering post-traumatic stress disorder (PTSD).

We also need to bear in mind that increasing numbers of fathers are reporting depression and PTSD following the birth of their children. They have in the past rarely discussed their feelings. However, the work of Mark Williams (2018) has raised awareness through his campaign Fathers Reaching Out.

Having a baby is a very intense and significant life-changing event. It is understandable that there is a normal emotional reaction to this change in circumstance. However, for some parents the emotional reaction can become more intense and difficult to manage and can aggravate pre-existing mental health issues.

Breastfeeding has been shown to offer some level of resilience to some mental health issues only if it is well supported (Borra et al. 2015). However, in our current economic crisis, support of breastfeeding can be lacking and inaccurate information leads to an increase in confusion, frustration and reduced breastfeeding rates. When mothers have stopped breastfeeding before they intended to they interpret this as a 'failure', the common phrase being 'I couldn't breastfeed my baby' or 'some women can't feed', which leaves the blame with the mother rather than lack of support from services and society.

As a result of this sense of failure, mothers can become self-critical and these negative thoughts can fuel any existing doubts that they are not doing well enough as a parent, leading to increasing anxiety and low mood. Breastfeeding does not fully protect against mental health issues but neither is it completely to blame for developing and maintaining them.

In a 2014 study (Figueiredo et al. 2014) showed that high depression scores in pregnancy tended to lead mothers either not to initiate breastfeeding, or to stop before 12 weeks. Although there may be many complicated factors as to why this could be the case, it suggests that mothers with depression may require extra support to establish and maintain breastfeeding.

As a health professional you play a key role in a family's access to health information and support. Ninety per cent of mental health issues are managed within primary care. The information you provide and advice you give have a significant impact on their decisions, especially if they are vulnerable and struggling to trust their own instincts and seeking reassurance and guidance. This can present difficulties if the situations are ones that you recall from your own days as a parent which you have not had the opportunity to de-brief. It is hard to promote breastfeeding if you feel that it was not right for you or indeed you also feel that you 'failed' to reach your own goals.

This chapter aims to identify some of the key issues which may occur for a breastfeeding mother with mental health issues and the importance of supporting her breastfeeding journey. There is not enough space to define every mental health issue that could occur during the perinatal or following period; however I have tried to identify, as a psychologist, some key features that may help you identify a mother who may be struggling and require additional support.

What issues might be difficult for mothers with depression or anxiety?

Rumination

This is churning over thoughts mentally, going over situations and comments repetitively. When our moods are negative then rumination becomes biased towards negative thoughts and predictions. Rumination is a failed problem-solving process. We get stuck in a loop, so the negative thoughts just go round and round without any solution.

The first remedy for rumination is to notice that it is happening. If mums notice a change in mood and that they are having an internal conversation with themselves this is a sign of rumination. Recognise that it is happening and that there is no purpose or solution with this mental activity, labelling it as rumination and making a decision to stop following this process. Secondly, we need to redirect the brain towards an engaging activity, possibly to feed mindfully and use this time to engage with the baby and the bond that is created through feeding – focusing on the sense of the baby's breathing and her own, which may be synchronised, looking at the fluttering of a baby's eyelids or the depth of the infant looking back at her, the clenching of fingers and toes as they relax.

Less time and ability to engage with normal stress-relieving activities

There are often activities that we develop which help us to relax and reconnect with our positive sense of self. Young babies, and some older ones as well, feed a lot and this may limit the freedom that a mother has to be away from her child to engage in enjoyable activities and hobbies outside the home. Consequently she has less access to activities which may normally help her maintain her mental wellbeing. This can lead to increased stress and also a loss of identity and social support. If a mum returns home to find a distressed and hungry baby and equally distressed partner who has been unable to settle the baby for the past 3 hours, she may not feel that the time out was worth the stress and may also feel guilty for trying to take time out for herself.

Problem solving may help the mother to adapt previously enjoyed activities to fit around breastfeeding, maybe at different times during the day when the baby is more settled with others, or for shorter periods of time which are more manageable between feeds.

Sleep

Lack of sleep can be a major trigger to feeling less emotionally resilient. Anxiety can also lead to mums struggling to rest when the baby sleeps. If worrying is becoming a significant problem, preventing a mum from sleeping, it may be worth considering whether she is presenting with generalised anxiety disorder (GAD).

Mothers may report that they are obsessively checking their baby for fear of cot death. This may be related to obsessive compulsive disorder and again, looking at some of the diagnostic criteria can be helpful to see whether mums are experiencing other symptoms.

If an anxiety disorder is suspected, a referral to a primary care mental health team for talking therapies may be appropriate or mothers can be signposted to online information to see if they relate to it.

If it is normal maternal exhaustion from waking through the night, then the common response is to suggest that bottles of expressed or formula milk are used to allow the partner to help with the night feeds. This may be helpful for some but often mothers still wake up when the baby cries, so sleep is still interrupted. It is also worth discussing with breastfeeding mothers that prolactin is at its highest production at night and stopping night feeds may impact on their milk supply. They may also risk blocked ducts and mastitis. Alternative options to help mothers reclaim some sleep may be partners taking babies first thing in the morning or during the evening so that the woman can rest.

Uncertainty and worry

Uncertainty is a significant trigger to anxiety and worry (Dugas and Roubichaud 1997). Worrying is characterised by a series of 'what if?' questions which tend to focus only on negative outcomes, and jump very quickly from one worry on to the next. These will often keep spiralling until they have reached a worst-case scenario. These 'what if?' questions and situations are normally future-based. Worry, similar to rumination, is a dysfunctional problem-solving strategy. It causes anxiety to build. It is worth reminding mothers that it is impossible to solve a situation which hasn't yet happened. The situation is imagined and may never happen.

Worrying can be the key characteristic of becoming a parent, but this may exacerbate any previous anxiety difficulties a mother has had. She may wish to address the wider issues through a talking therapy. However, worry is also something that most people do in uncertain situations and babies are a very uncertain factor in life.

With worry we need to step away from the hypothetical situations and focus on the real problem if there is one. If there is a real problem then we can work on solving it. You cannot solve a problem that has not yet happened. For example, a mother may be struggling with poor attachment and perceived milk supply. She may be worrying that if this doesn't get resolved she won't produce enough milk, the baby will lose weight and will have to be readmitted to hospital. In the extreme situation the baby may get seriously ill. At this stage switching to formula milk may seem the best option. However, if the baby is gaining weight these are hypothetical issues. The real problem may be that the attachment is not effective or that she is not responding to baby's cues to feed such that her milk supply may not be stimulated. That is something she can work on with a breastfeeding expert. You may plan to review mother and baby if you are satisfied that the baby is not at risk and will be monitored by another health professional. Help the mum also to stay focused more around the present, by focusing on getting through the next feed and the next day rather than trying to plan for the next week or focusing on exclusive feeding for 6 months. Smaller goals will feel more achievable and lead to a greater sense of control which helps to build confidence. Support families with the information that every breastfeed they achieve is positive and any breastfeeding has benefits for her baby. Encourage them to stay in the present. Again, using mindful feeding may be helpful to focus on one feed at a time, one day at a time.

How can breastfeeding support mental wellbeing?

Breastfeeding produces oxytocin which encourages emotional attachments and a sense of calmness. This may also help mothers settle into the change in their situation from possibly a role in management to becoming a new mother with little control or routine.

- Oxytocin aids sleep by allowing mothers to fall asleep again faster and by reversing the effects of cortisol (Uvnäs Moberg and Odent 2011).
- Breastfeeding mothers are more likely to co-sleep with babies which can lead to less interrupted sleep patterns.
- Although breastfeeding can initially have its own challenges, it requires less practical planning, in the sense of preparing formula. For a mother who may be struggling with motivation and energy to manage housework tasks this reduces stress.
- If breastfeeding is a key value for a mother then being able to engage in this activity leads to her feeling more engaged in her parenting goals and positive, affirming behaviours.

Mental health in the perinatal period and breastfeeding

The 'baby blues' are experienced by many parents. The sudden changes in hormones and realisation of having a baby to care for can feel overwhelming and lead mothers to become tearful, anxious and low for a few days after birth. If we add physical recovery and pain from the recent birth along with lack of sleep it is understandable that this is a difficult period. This emotional state normally starts to resolve itself within the first few weeks after birth as parents gain more experience and confidence. However, as previously discussed, babies bring with them a significant increase in uncertainty and responsibility as well as a change in social circumstance, all of which

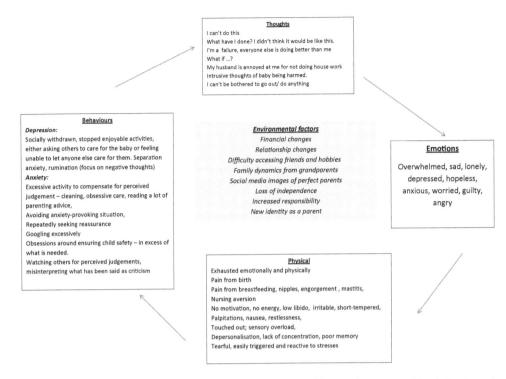

Figure 10.1 Thoughts, feelings and behaviours experienced by mothers – cognitive behavioural therapy (CBT) model

Source: Williams and Garland (2002).

are significant vulnerability factors for developing a mental health problem or exacerbating a pre-existing one.

To help illustrate some the issues that might be happening during the perinatal period I have used a basic cognitive behavioural therapy (CBT) (Williams and Garland 2002) model in Figure 10.1.

This diagram separates the potential symptoms and triggers into easily graspable sections and how they may impact on one another. A mother may experience some or all of these symptoms or more.

If a significant number of these are present for over a month then this is an indication that a mental health issue may be developing and support should be offered. To support discussions around difficulties the Patient Health Questionnaire (PHQ9) and Generalised Anxiety Disorder (GAD7) should be used. These rate the frequency of symptoms over the past 2 weeks and can be used as a discussion point and severity rating for mood. These are freely available on the internet and are also used within mental health teams so may be useful when making referrals.

How to support a breastfeeding mother with a mental health issue

Often when a breastfeeding mother reports depression or anxiety she is met with well-intended sentiments related to her breastfeeding, such as 'no one would blame you if you stopped', 'maybe you need to look after yourself now' or 'if you use a bottle then others can help out'.

These phrases may all be true. A mother may need to start considering how she looks after her own mental wellbeing, she may need to access some support from others with childcare, and no one should blame her if she chooses to change how she is feeding her child. However, all these comments imply that the breastfeeding is to blame for the mental health issues. It implies that by stopping or reducing breastfeeding then her mood will resolve, or that looking after herself is mutually exclusive from continuing to breastfeed.

Breastfeeding may be perceived as a drain on the mother. In truth, any way of feeding a baby has its own level of demands, restrictions and commitments. However, don't blame the breastfeeding for mental health issues. As we can see from Figure 10.1, there are a significant number of elements within a parenting relationship which affect our mood; breastfeeding is just one of them and for mothers it may not be a negative one.

Breastfeeding as a core belief value

Attitudes to breastfeeding vary between people. Some are fairly ambivalent to breastfeeding, believing breastfeeding and formula to be equal. Others passionately believe in breastfeeding and will avoid using any substitute at all costs. There is an array in between. Stopping breastfeeding before they planned may affect each of these women differently. For the ambivalent being given advice to top up with formula or suggesting they stop or reduce breastfeeding may be met with little resistance or emotional turmoil. However, for some women breastfeeding – the physical, emotional and nutritional element of nurturing their baby – may be very deeply important to them. It may have been part of the imagery they had before becoming a mother, something they researched or may have been an important part of feeding previous children. For them it has become a core parenting value which has a significant importance and meaning.

Most psychosocial models of mental health focus on stable mental health being based around engaging in activities which are meaningful to the patient (e.g. CBT (Lejuez et al. 2011), acceptance and commitment therapy (ACT) (Hayes et al. 2011), dialectical behavioural therapy (DBT) (Lineham 2015). The life (in this case parenting) values that we each hold are individual. By focusing on these and engaging with them, patients increase the number of positive and self-affirming activities which then enable greater thought balancing and positive mood. It also provides a sense of living our lives in accordance with our values and gives a sense of achievement and enjoyment.

If breastfeeding is an important value, removing it can lead to a significant feeling of failure, loss and guilt. Alongside these emotions intense negative and self-critical thoughts lead to greater levels of depression and anxiety. Many breastfeeding mothers report that they do not wish to speak to health professionals about their mental health for fear that they will be told to stop and the importance of breastfeeding to them dismissed.

Supporting mothers who wish to continue breastfeeding

If a mother with mental health issues wishes to breastfeed and it is safe for her and her baby, every support should be given to allow them to continue.

Many mothers report that the comments of health professionals can have a significant impact on how they feel about their feeding journey. Some mothers have reported feeling under pressure to breastfeed and judged if they chose to stop. Others felt that their desire to continue breastfeeding was undermined and seen as selfish or unnecessary. As a health professional the power balance between you and the mother is tipped in your direction. You are perceived as knowledgeable and skilled. Your advice is taken to heart and can influence the decisions that a mother then makes. This is especially true when a mother may have mental health difficulties and is struggling to trust her own judgement or problem solve a situation. At this time, she may be seeking reassurance, desperate for solutions. Meanwhile she is lacking in confidence to challenge decisions she may not feel are right for her and her baby. It is important to ensure that you are giving evidence-based information to enable an informed decision rather than a personal opinion on the situation. If you do not have a relevant knowledge or experience about breastfeeding, then signpost the family to breastfeeding support services. This enables the mother to be empowered to make an informed decision about how she feeds her baby.

Many women are not aware that their symptoms may be related to low mood or anxiety and may report somatised symptoms instead; these include low energy, feeling exhausted but unable to sleep, racing mind and heart palpitations. Mothers may also seek repeated reassurance around their own or the baby's health or appear overly anxious about decisions.

If a mother is presenting with these issues, exploring whether she may be suffering from other difficulties with mood can be helpful. Many parents can be reluctant to acknowledge difficulties due to the stigma of mental health or fear that if they say they are struggling their children will be taken away. Others may be unaware that the difficulties they are facing may be part of a wider picture, and something that they could get support with.

As a health worker you may not have experience or the resources in your service to be able to provide specific support for mental health needs, but helping them to recognise what may be happening with their mood and signposting them to where they can get support can be essential in the first steps to managing mental health issues.

There is a list of useful websites and self-help materials at the end of this chapter. Allowing mothers to explore the symptoms and decide for themselves whether they feel support may be relevant to them is far more empowering then just being told you are depressed or anxious which can lead to feeling dismissed.

Supporting mothers who decide to stop feeding

Some mothers may feel that being solely reliant for feeding their baby or overcoming any breastfeeding difficulties they are facing is too overwhelming for them and they may decide that they wish to stop or look at alternative feeding methods. If this is the best decision for them to be able to maintain their own mental wellbeing then we should support their right to make the decision and praise them for any breastfeeding they have achieved.

Many mothers report that they feel they failed and that health professionals judged them for formula feeding. Reinforce that if they are making decisions that they need to look after themselves and this is the right decision for them, then that is fine. It may also be important at this point to acknowledge any feelings of loss or guilt that a mother may feel through this decision, however old the child is. Breastfeeding is a relationship between mother and child which has a biological impact on how they react to each other. When this ends there may for some mothers be a sense of bereavement at the loss of this relationship or guilt that it is their decision to end it. There are not problem-solving solutions to this emotion, but listening and acknowledging how they feel allows them space to process this.

Mothers may also need additional support around the process of stopping feeding as babies may not always initially take a bottle and it may reinforce the guilt if babies are getting distressed when feeding. They also needs to be awareness of the potential need to express or slowly reduce feeding to prevent engorgement or mastitis so self-care during this time is very important.

If mothers stopped breastfeeding before they wanted to with previous children but wish to try again with subsequent babies, it may be useful to work through a 'debrief' during pregnancy to look at where they encountered problems last time and what they and the services around them can put in place to maybe make them more successful with future children. This may include thinking about self-care and emotional support to help manage difficulties whilst establishing feeding, or at times when they found it more demanding.

Talking therapies

Some mothers do not wish to take antidepressants and would prefer to explore other treatment options. Talking therapies and in particular CBT are recommended by the National Institute for Health and Care Excellence (NICE) (CG 192, NICE 2014; Royal College of General Practitioners 2015) for depression and anxiety disorders. Most services will prioritise mothers (and sometimes fathers) in the perinatal period for therapy; however, it is worth noting that not all services allow women to bring their babies to therapy sessions. This is due to two reasons. Firstly, therapy should be a focused change intervention which requires a client to concentrate throughout the session. As any parent will attest, nothing interferes with your concentration more than a child. This is true for both mother and therapist. It is very difficult to conduct an in-depth discussion with a mother on her core negative thoughts when there is a baby in the room giggling or crying. Secondly, with regard to older children, they become more aware of mother's emotional state and if she is processing something in a session and becomes emotional, this can then lead to the child or toddler becoming distressed. Mothers in turn then to try and shut these emotions down, which leads to limited effect during the session.

Parents may need to find childcare support for their sessions. If sessions are located away from home and young babies are breastfed it is worth exploring whether someone can care for the baby outside of the session room but nearby. If the baby needs to be breastfed the carer can have bring the baby to the mother or the mother can step out briefly. Although this may still cause some disruption to the sessions, it may be better than the mother not being able to access any support in this critical period.

With most NHS mental health services being run on a weekday 9 a.m. to 5 p.m. service, childcare may present barriers. An increasing number of services are starting to run sessions outside of these hours but these may be delivered via other means such as by telephone or online services rather than face to face.

As mentioned, therapy is a change process so mothers also need to be able to process what they are working on in between sessions. Even if they do not wish to engage in therapy sessions, an assessment with a team may still be useful as they can advise and signpost a mother towards self-help support or psychoeducation to help manage her condition until the time feels right for her to work on treatment sessions.

Summary

- If a mother is anxious or depressed she is vulnerable. What you say can have a huge impact on her mood, even from unintentional subtle cues from body language.
- If a mother wishes to continue breastfeeding her baby she should be given all the support available to allow her to continue to do so. If breastfeeding is an important parenting value for her, supporting her to continue will enable her to engage with her personal value system which in turn helps manage her mood.
- Mothers with depression and anxiety are less likely to maintain breastfeeding beyond 3 months. They may require additional emotional support in the early weeks whilst feeding becomes established.
- Support mothers to engage with preferred stress-reducing activities whilst maintaining breastfeeding as they wish.
- If a mother wishes to combi feed (use a mixture of breast and bottlefeeding) or to stop breastfeeding, support her to do so whilst avoiding mastitis. Acknowledge how she may feel about the decision to stop. Breastfeeding is a relationship and some mothers feel a bereavement at the loss of this element of parenting. Referral to a breastfeeding specialist may be appropriate.
- Offer alternatives to medication where appropriate. Although antidepressants are safe to take during lactation, some mothers may prefer not to take these and may wish to access talking therapies instead.
- Do not generalise all emotional difficulties as postnatal depression – there are many other common mental health disorders which may occur within this period, e.g. PTSD, obsessive compulsive disorder, anxiety.
- Provide mothers with evidence-based information to allow them to make an informed decision about how they manage their mental wellbeing alongside feeding their child. Whatever decisions they make, support them to maintain their mental wellbeing.

Self-help resources

- Anxiety UK: www.anxietyuk.org.uk
- Birth Trauma Association: www.birthtraumaassociation.org.uk/
- Centre for Clinical Interventions (self-help workbooks and information sheets): www.cci.health.wa.gov.au/Resources/Looking-After-Yourself
- Exeter Worry Management Guide: https://cedar.exeter.ac.uk/media/university ofexeter/schoolofpsychology/cedar/documents/Worry_website_version_colour.pdf
- Fathers Reaching Out: www.reachingoutpmh.co.uk/daddy-blues-by-mark-williams/
- Get Self Help (self-help guides and information sheets): www.getselfhelp.co.uk

- Maternal OCD: https://maternalocd.org/
- MIND: www.mind.org.uk
- Northumberland mental health guides: https://web.ntw.nhs.uk/selfhelp/

References

Borra C, Iacovou M, Sevilla A (2015) New evidence on breastfeeding and postpartum depression: the importance of understanding women's intentions. *Matern Child Health J* 19(4):897–907.

Dugas MJ, Roubichaud M (1997) *Cognitive-behavioural Treatment of Generalised Anxiety Disorder. From Science to Practice.* New York: Routledge.

Figueiredo B, Canario C, Field T (2014) Breastfeeding is negatively affected by prenatal depression and reduces postpartum depression. *Psychol Med* 44:927–936.

Hayes SC, Strosahl KD, Wilson KG (2011) *Acceptance and Commitment Therapy: The Process and Practice of Mindful Change.* Guilford Press.

Lejuez CW, Hopko DR, Acierno R, Daughters SB, Pagoto SL (2011) Ten year revision of the brief behavioural activation treatment for depression: revised treatment manual. *Behav Modification* 35(2):111–161.

Linehan M (2015) *DBT Skills Training Manual.* Guilford Press.

NICE (2014) *Antenatal and Postnatal Mental Health: Clinical Management and Service Guidance.* NICE guidelines (CG192). www.nice.org.uk/guidance/CG192

Royal College of General Practitioners (2015) *Practical Implications for Primary Care of the NICE guidelines CG192.* http://tvscn.nhs.uk/wp-content/uploads/2015/07/RCGP-Ten-Top-Tips-Nice-Guidance-June-2015.ashx_.pdf

Uvnäs Moberg K, Odent M (2011) *The Oxytocin Factor: Tapping the Hormone of Calm, Love and Healing.* Pinter and Martin.

Williams C, Garland A (2002) A cognitive-behavioural therapy assessment model for use in everyday clinical practice. *Adv Psychiatric Treat* 8:172–179.

Williams M (2018) *Daddy Blues. Postnatal Depression and Fatherhood.* Trigger.

11 Tongue tie

Sarah Oakley

- Ankyloglossia, also known as tongue tie, is a congenital anomaly characterised by an abnormally short lingual frenulum; the tip of the tongue cannot be protruded beyond the lower incisor teeth. It varies in degree, from a mild form in which the tongue is bound only by a thin mucous membrane to a severe form in which the tongue is completely fused to the floor of the mouth.
- Throughout history there has been a tendency to dismiss tongue tie as a fabrication and to question under what circumstances tongue ties should be divided and by whom. What we know is that a lingual frenulum is normal anatomy so when assessing infants with feeding issues in relation to potential tongue tie the focus needs to be on tongue function.
- Evidence-based tools are available to help on this process. But advanced infant feeding knowledge and experience are also required to exclude and address other factors which may be contributing to the feeding difficulties. In this way we can ensure that only those babies who are most likely to benefit are treated.

There are few more controversial issues in infant feeding than tongue tie. Tongue tie and its impact on infant feeding are dogged by misinformation, misunderstanding, denial and conflicting ideas. This is compounded by poor education amongst healthcare professionals and some breastfeeding supporters.

But the controversy is not new, nor is the idea that tongue ties can cause problems and require treatment. Cullum (1959) in an article in the *British Medical Journal* explores the history of tongue tie through the medical literature and describes his own experience of observing this 'little operation' with 'dramatic' results in infants who were struggling to bottlefeed. Cullum cites *The Nurses' Guide, or the Right Method of Bringing Up Young Children,* by 'an eminent physician', published in London in 1729: 'Very often the membrane under the tongue is so short and strait that it hinders the child from sucking'. He also reports this observation by William Moss, a Liverpool surgeon from 1794:

> A child's being tongue-tied will impede and hinder his sucking freely. When that happens he may be observed to lose his hold very often, and when he draws the breast he frequently makes a chucking noise. Upon this ocassion the mouth must

be examined and the tongue set at liberty by cutting the ligament or string which will be found to confine the tongue down to the lower part of the mouth and which is done by the surgeon with little or no pain to the child who will commonly take the breast immediately after the operation ... One out of three or four childen are tongue-tied more or less.

(Cullum 1959)

But it was not only surgeons who were reported to be dividing tongue ties during the 18th century. In 1764, John Theobald (cited by Cullum 1959) wrote, 'it may be necessary to cut the bridle of the tongue and this is usually done by nurses and midwives with their nail'. Nils Rosen von Rosenstein, Swedish Royal Physician, 1776 wrote:

When children do not work well our old women say that they are tongue-tied and pretend that the bridle ought to be snipped with a pair of scissors. I have never as yet seen any child's tongue tied ... should an operation be judged necessary for it ought never be done with the nails but performed by some experienced man, otherwise one of the blood vessels near the tongue might easily be opened.

(Cullum 1959)

Controversy over who should divide tongue ties and the idea that the condition is a fabrication persist today. Many NHS trusts are of the view that the procedure should only be carried out by surgeons, despite the large number of midwives and nurses who have been trained and perform this procedure (who are arguably much better placed to provide such a service if they also have advance specialist skills in infant feeding). National Institute for Health and Care Excellence (NICE) guidance (2005) states division should be performed by registered healthcare professionals, not specifically surgeons. An article published in the Australian *Sunday Telegraph* (Hansen 2016) reports, 'Doctors are warning that, in most cases, the issue naturally heals over time and the rapid rise [in division] is a fad'. The article goes on to quote the opinions of two surgeons which reflect this. In contrast, Messner and Lalakea (2000) found that, whilst 69% of lactation consultants believed tongue tie is associated with feeding problems, only a minority of physicians did. The controversy seems to be exacerbated by the fact that, whilst tongue tie itself is a feeding issue in infants and so falls within the remit of midwives, health visitors, nurses and lactation consultants, division is a surgical procedure and so crosses over into the world of the medical profession.

All healthcare professionals are duty-bound by their codes of conduct to provide evidence-based information and base their decisions on the best evidence available.

The vast majority of humans are thought to have a lingual frenulum (a membrane situated towards the base of the tongue which extends from the undersurface of the tongue into the floor of the mouth) (Figure 11.1) so the presence of a visible or palpable lingual frenulum is normal anatomy and not in itself an indication that division is required (Haham et al. (2014) found that 199/200 babies had a visible or palpable lingual frenulum). However, in some individuals this lingual frenulum may be short, tight and attached close to the tip of the tongue and/or on the gum, causing restrictions in tongue movement and function. These restricted lingual frenula may then cause feeding difficulties and are what we call a 'tongue tie' (or ankyloglossia).

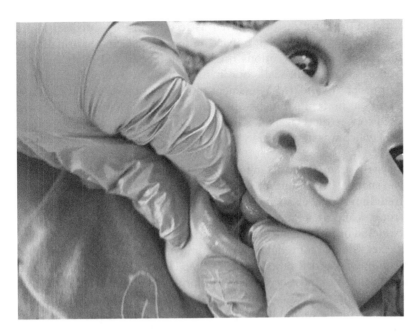

Figure 11.1 Examination of frenulum
Source: © S. Oakley with permission.

Incidence rates have been cited by Francis et al. (2015) at between 0.2% and 10.7%. However, they and many others have acknowledged the difficulties in obtaining accurate incidence data due to a lack of agreement on diagnostic criteria.

An Australian study published by Todd and Hogan (2015) reported a division rate for early feeding issues of 4.7–5.0% in their combined sample of over 5,000 babies. In contrast, Martinelli et al. (2015) reported that 14 babies from a sample of 109 underwent division, providing a higher rate of division of 12%. Again division rates will vary depending on the diagnostic criteria used for identifying tongue tie, the level of infant feeding support available, infant factors such as prematurity and the presence of abnormalities and developmental issues, maternal factors such as pain tolerance, milk supply, previous breastfeeding experience and the acceptability of the procedure to parents.

It is easy to see, given that a lingual frenulum is normal anatomy, that there is a risk of overdiagnosis, which is why a thorough feeding assessment and assessment of tongue function are needed by a professional who has extensive knowledge and training in infant feeding and tongue-tie division. This is currently not happening in many services, as reflected in the huge variations in services found in a survey conducted by the National Childbirth Trust (NCT) (Wise 2015).

Tongue tie is caused by incomplete normal tissue degeneration (apoptosis) during the embryological formation period of the tongue. Both genetic and environmental factors are believed to influence this incomplete apoptosis (Hazelbaker 2010). The abnormal metabolism of folic acid linked to the *MTHFR* gene mutation has been proposed as a factor, but a review of the literature reveals that there is no published evidence to support this theory currently.

Assessment of tongue tie involves taking a thorough history, including the maternal and infant medical history, birth history as well as feeding history. Medical issues such as maternal endocrine disorders can impact on feeding, as can abnormality or prematurity in the infant and interventions used during labour and birth. Feeding should be observed to assess latch, seal, coordination of suck/swallow/breathe and efficiency of milk transfer. A validated assessment tool should then be used to assess tongue tie which looks at both function as well as appearance. The most well-known and frequently used tool is the Hazelbaker Assessment Tool for Lingual Frenulum Function (HATLFF) which was developed by American lactation consultant Dr Alison Hazelbaker in 1993.

The tool consists of seven function items – extension, elevation, lateralisation, cupping, peristalsis, snapback and anterior spread – and five appearance items – tongue tip appearance, frenulum length, elasticity of frenulum, attachment of frenulum to the undersurface of tongue and attachment to the gum/floor of the mouth. Hazelbaker observed 3,000 babies in order to define what constitutes a restricted lingual frenulum and the tool has been evaluated for reliability and validity (Amir et al. 2006). This tool is complex, and training is needed in its use. However, Hazelbaker has trademarked it so any teaching on this tool must be done by her or a trainer approved by her. As a result formal training opportunities are limited but she has a detailed section in her book (2010) on the use of the tool and it is possible to learn how to use it through observation of those who have been trained.

An updated version of the HATLFF can be accessed via www.alisonhazelbaker. com/shop.

A simpler tool derived from the HATLFF is the Bristol Tongue Assessment Tool (Ingram 2015). This tool consists of four items – tongue tip appearance, attachment of frenulum to lower gum ridge, lift of tongue with mouth wide (crying) and tongue protrusion. It requires minimal training and experience to use and for professionals involved in supporting mothers and babies is a useful tool for identifying potential tongue tie. It has been adopted in areas such as Kent for use by their health visiting staff. A visual version of this tool is now available, called the TABBY Assessment Tool, which will make this tool even more accessible (www.bristol.ac.uk/academic-child-health/research/research/childdevelopmentdisability/tongue-tie/).

The tool is scored out of 8, with a score of 0–3 indicative of the more severe type of tongue tie. I suggest that all babies scoring 6 or below should be referred to a practitioner with infant feeding and tongue-tie expertise for more detailed assessment before a decision to divide is made.

In some cases where a tongue tie has been identified, restriction in function will be severe and the associated feeding issues will be acute. It will be easy to relate tongue-tie function to the symptoms being seen (Table 11.1).

However, in other cases of milder tongue restriction, particularly when this coexists alongside other issues such as a high or bubble palate, a history of birth trauma, jaw tension, plagiocephaly, torticollis, prematurity, low birthweight and other infant health issues, it can be difficult to ascertain the degree to which the tongue tie is impacting on infant feeding and predict the outcome of a division. In all cases of tongue tie attention needs to be paid to improving positioning and attachment and milk transfer through strategies such as breast compression, switch nursing and increasing supply. But in the cases of milder restriction these types of conservative approaches, alongside interventions such as cranial osteopathy, chiropractic, physiotherapy and speech

Table 11.1 Restriction in tongue function

Restriction in tongue function	Symptoms
Inability to extend tongue over bottom lip	Nipple pain and damage Inability to latch Difficulty latching Difficulty sustaining the latch (baby slips down or off the breast)
Inability to lift the tongue to mid-mouth or above	Inefficient feeding – long feeds, frequent feeds, slow weight gain, weight loss Flow regulation issues – coughing and choking at the breast, tiring at the breast
Inability to cup the breast securely	Difficulty sustaining the latch (baby slips down or off the breast) Loss of suction (clicking) Difficulty forming a seal (dribbling during feeds) Aerophagia contributing to abdominal pain and reflux
Inability to keep the tongue in a forward position (snapback)	Slipping off the breast Clicking sounds during feeding
Inability to form a peristaltic wave with the tongue	Inefficient feeding due to insufficient vacuum to transfer milk – high suck-to-swallow ratio, tiring, long or frequent feeds, weight issues

and language therapy input may yield significant improvements without the need for a division. Studies looking at the use of osteopathy and chiropractic include those by Miller (2009) and Wescott (2004).

Treatment of tongue tie

The procedure used most commonly to divide a restricted frenulum in an infant (Figure 11.2) is a frenulotomy, as per NICE guidance (2005). This technique involves swaddling the baby, holding the head still, lifting the tongue and dividing the lingual frenulum with scissors. (Laser is an alternative but is only available privately in the UK and the added expense has not proven as worthwhile in terms of outcomes.) The procedure is not thought to be painful due to the absence of nerves within the frenulum and anecdotal reports, so local anaesthetic is not generally used. A case series of 215 babies found that 18% slept through the procedure and only 1% cried for more than a minute (Griffiths 2004). Babies are fed immediately afterwards and this calms them, stems bleeding and if they are breastfed the endorphins in the breastmilk will help soothe any discomfort (Shah et al. 2012).

Risks include bleeding, damage to other structures in the mouth, infection and recurrence. Bleeding is usually minimal. An unpublished audit by the Association

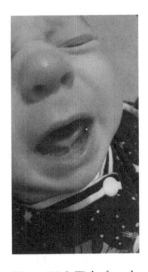

Figure 11.2 Tight frenulum before cutting
Source: © S. Oakley with permission.

of Tongue-tie Practitioners in 2018 collected data from 50 practitioners who had carried out approximately 77,000 procedures. Most of these babies stopped bleeding within a few minutes whilst feeding. One in 7,000 required the use of adrenaline and only one out of the 77,000 required cautery. Guidelines on managing bleeding post-frenulotomy can be found here: www.tongue-tie.org.uk/wp-content/uploads/2019/08/Guideline-for-the-management-of-bleeding-post-frenulotomy-2019v1.pdf.

The risk of bleeding can be mitigated by checking for family history of bleeding disorders and ensuring baby has had vitamin K at birth. The risk posed by not having vitamin K is difficult to quantify and frenulotomy is performed on babies who have not had vitamin K in some instances after a risk assessment and with informed choice of the parents. A clotting screen may be done in such cases prior to division.

Infection after division is very rare and, based on data from the Wessex Tongue-tie Service (www.uhs.nhs.uk/OurServices/Childhealth/Tonguetie/Tonguetie.aspx), is said to be less than one in 10,000. Any infection usually responds well to antibiotics. There has been one serious case reported in 2010 where a baby succumbed to an infection caused by *Klebsiella oxytoca*.

It is entirely normal for the wound to form a white scab resembling a mouth ulcer as it heals, and this scab usually resolves within 7–14 days and it not a sign of infection. In jaundiced babies the scab may look yellow/orange.

Damage to other structures in the mouth is also rare and should be minimised with care and training. The author has seen a case where the submandibular glands were damaged causing a localised swelling in the mouth which resolved after several weeks without treatment. Cases of similar damage have been reported in the USA and may require surgical intervention.

Recurrence of tongue tie is the most common complication we see and most controversial. Allegations are made of inadequate division, but all practitioners will have some recurrences and there are conflicting opinions on what constitutes a full release, although a visible diamond-shaped wound is what most practitioners aim for. The most common cause of recurrence is thought to be due to scarring, with thicker frenula appearing to have more of a tendency for this. Histology studies done in Brazil (Martinelli and Marcheson 2014) found that the thicker frenula are higher in collagen and more tendon-like in structure than the thinner types, which would explain why the more posterior-type tongue ties, which are often quite thick, seem more prone to recurrence.

Claims are made by some authorities that disrupting the wound during healing through repeated massage or stretching reduces the risk of recurrence but there is no published evidence to support this approach and there are concerns regarding the risk of bleeding, infection and pain. Cases of oral aversion have been reported and parents are reluctant to do it due to the distress caused to the baby. Unpublished data collected by the Association of Tongue-tie Practitioners indicates an average second division rate of 3–4%, so numbers are low.

Parents should be made aware that some babies can be quite unsettled after the procedure and feeding may deteriorate before it gets better. For some babies the freedom of tongue movement seems to be confusing and those who have been very restricted often struggle with low muscle tone in the first few days and may find feeding tiring. Occasionally babies will refuse to latch in the first few days after division. In all cases it is imperative that parents have access to skilled follow-up help and support.

The efficacy of tongue-tie division is often called into question and many of the medical profession have the impression that there is no research to support the use of frenulotomy as an intervention to support breastfeeding, despite the NICE guidance (2005). Some of the published papers on this issue include Hogan et al. (2005), Buryk et al. (2011), Edmunds et al. (2011), Berry et al. (2012), Finnigan and Long (2013), O'Callahan et al. (2013), Emond (2014), Ito (2014), Ghaheri et al. (2017) and Ramoser et al. (2019).

Of course, as with any surgical intervention, the procedure itself may be successful but that does not guarantee a successful outcome. What is lacking in the existing research is long-term follow-up and outcomes. Ethically it is difficult to withhold an intervention which seems to have some benefits from a control group and in the published studies most of the babies in the control group were offered and had division shortly after it became clear that improvements were being seen in the intervention groups. Most studies have only followed up on short-term outcomes. Again, there are difficulties in attributing long-term outcomes to the procedure because there are so many factors influencing successful breastfeeding outcomes. Delays in diagnosis and treatment of tongue tie may result in loss of confidence in the mother, poor weight gain, low milk supply and supplementation with formula which will all shorten the duration of breastfeeding. Furthermore, access to skilled ongoing breastfeeding support is not universally available and healthcare professional education in infant feeding is inconsistent. Social pressures in terms of family support, the need to return to work, how breastfeeding is portrayed in the media and so on will all influence how long a mother breastfeeds. So, outcomes are not simply going to be related to frenulotomy.

The issue of tongue tie in relation to infant feeding has, as discussed, always been controversial and remains so at the current time. However, those of us working with families affected by tongue tie and who provide frenulotomy do see improvements in feeding from this intervention in most cases. The focus must be on identifying those dyads most likely to benefit from tongue-tie division and ensuring they have access to timely and skilled support.

Ultimately, we need to listen to the parents and work with them, keeping an open mind, to find satisfactory solutions to their breastfeeding difficulties.

References

Amir L, James J, Donath S (2006) Reliability of the Hazelbaker assessment tool for lingual frenulum function. *Int Breastfeed J* 1:3.

Berry J, Griffiths M, Westcott C (2012) A double-blind, randomised controlled trial of tongue-tie division and its immediate effect on breastfeeding. *Breastfeed Med* 7:189–93.

Buryk M, Bloom D, Shope T (2011) Efficacy of neonatal release of ankyloglossia: a randomized trial. *Pediatrics* 128:280–6.

Cullum IM (1959) An old wive's tale. *Br Med J* 2:498

Edmunds J, Miles S, Fulbrook P (2011) Tongue-tie and breastfeeding: a review of the literature. *Breastfeed Rev* 19(1):19–26.

Emond A (2014) Randomised controlled trial of early frenotomy in breastfed infants with mild–moderate tongue-tie. *Arch Dis Child – Fetal Neonat Ed* 99:F189–95.

Finnigan V, Long T (2013) The effectiveness of frenulotomy on infant feeding outcomes: a systematic review. *Evid Based Midwif* 11(2):40–5.

Francis DO, Krishnaswami S, McPheeters M (2015) Treatment of ankyloglossia and breastfeeding outcomes: a systematic review. *Pediatrics* 135(6):1458–66.

Ghaheri B, Cole M, Fausel S, Chuop M, Mace J (2017) Breastfeeding improvement following tongue-tie and lip-tie release: a prospective cohort study. *Laryngoscope* 127(5):1217–23.

Griffiths DM (2004) Do tongue-ties affect breastfeeding? *J Hum Lactat* 20:409–14,

Haham A, Mangel L, Marom R, Botzer E (2014) Prevalence of breastfeeding difficulties in newborns with a lingual frenulum: a prospective cohort series. *Breastfeed Med* 9(9):438–41.

Hansen J (2016) Doctors warning parents to stop new fad of operating on their baby's tongues. *Sunday Telegraph*. www.dailytelegraph.com.au/news/doctors-warning-parents-to-stop-new-fad-of-operating-on-their-babys-tongues/news-story/bdc5a7fe78e74da01b3290d85ab14655

Hazelbaker A (2010) *Tongue-tie: Morphogenesis, Impact, Assessment and Treatment.* Aidan and Eva Press.

Hogan M, Westcott C, Griffiths M (2005) A randomised, controlled trial of division of tongue-tie in infants with feeding problems. *J Paediatr Child Health* 41(5–6):246–50.

Ingram J, Johnson D, Copeland M, Churchill C, Taylor H, Emond A (2015) The development of a tongue assessment tool to assist with tongue-tie identification. *Arch Dis Child: Fetal Neonat Ed* 100(4):F344–9.

Ito Y (2014) Does frenotomy improve breast-feeding difficulties in infants with ankyloglossia? *Pediatr Int* 56:497.

Martinelli R, Marcheson I (2014) Histological characteristics of altered human lingual frenulum. *Int J Pediatr Child Health* 2:5–9.

Martinelli R, Marchesan IQ, Gusmao RJ, Honorio HM, Berretin-Felix G (2015) The effects of frenotomy on breastfeeding. *J Appl Oral Sci* 23(2):153–7.

Messner AH, Lalakea ML (2000) Ankyloglossia: controversies in management. *Int J Pediatr Otorhinolaryngol* 54(2–3):123–31.

Miller JE (2009) Contribution of chiropractic therapy to resolving suboptimal breastfeeding: a case series of 114 infants. *J Manipulative Physiol Ther* 32(8):670–4.

NICE (2005) *Division of ankyloglossia (tongue-tie) for breastfeeding* IPG 149. www.nice.org.uk/guidance/ipg149

O'Callahan C, Macary S, Clemente S (2013) The effects of office-based frenotomy for anterior and posterior ankyloglossia on breastfeeding. *Int J Pediatr Otorhinolaryngol* 77:827–32.

Ramoser G, Guoth-Gumberger M, Baumgartner-Sigl S, Zoeggeler T, Scholl-Burgi S, Karall D (2019) Frenotomy for tongue-tie (frenulum linguae breve) showed improved symptoms in the short- and long-term follow-up. *Acta Paediatr* doi: 10.1111/apa.14811 [epub ahead of print].

Shah PS, Herbozo C, Aliwalas LL, Shah VS (2012) Breastfeeding or breast milk for procedural pain in neonates. *Cochrane Database of Systematic Reviews* (12).

Todd DA, Hogan MJ (2015) Tongue-tie in the newborn: early diagnosis and division prevents poor breastfeeding outcomes. *Breastfeed Rev* 23(1):11–16.

Wescott N (2004) The use of cranial osteopathy in the treatment of infants with breast feeding problems or sucking dysfunction. *Aust J Holist Nurs* 11(1):25–32.

Wise P (2015) Huge variations in NHS infant tongue-tie services NCT, 2016. www.nct.org.uk/sites/default/files/related_documents/Wise%20Huge%20variation%20in%20NHS%20infant%20tongue-tie%20services.pdf

12 Colic and reflux in the breastfed baby

Shel Banks

Exclusive breastfeeding is the best form of nutrition for infants under 6 months of age, and this should be promoted, supported and protected wherever possible – do not suggest that breastfeeding should stop to manage colic, reflux or other allergy symptoms.

Specialist milks and medications should only be considered when there is truly a clinical need after a thorough assessment.

Assessment should include an appropriately skilled and experienced person looking at common feeding management issues, and consideration of whether the appropriate infant feed products are being prepared, stored and fed to baby correctly.

Note: Colic and reflux are separate symptoms.

Infantile colic

The term infantile colic was defined in 1954 by paediatrician Dr Morris Wessel as a minimum of 3 hours' crying per day, for a minimum of 3 days in a week, for 3 weeks between the third week and third month of life: the so-called 'Rule of 3' (Wessel et al. 1954) Typically, we see a baby where crying is in excess of a normal range of distress, with inconsolable crying; classically, there is a very high-pitched cry, and the parents will be exhausted and frustrated. The paroxysms of inconsolable crying are often accompanied by what appear to be gut-related symptoms: flushing of the face, clenching of fists, arching of the back, meteorism, drawing up of the legs and flatulence (Savino and Tarasco 2010).

A more modern definition from the Rome IV criteria abandons the 'Rule of 3' (Koppen et al. 2017), and new definitions include the phrase 'spasmodic contraction of the smooth wall of the intestine, causing pain and discomfort', which makes sense to us as observers, understanding the gut involvement.

Symptoms have historically typically started in the second week of life in both breastfed and formula-fed infants and resolved by 3 months of age (Lucas and St James-Roberts 1998). Generally speaking, these symptoms are not indicative of disease and so seeking medical attention for these infants is generally unnecessary, may be detrimental and should not be encouraged (Savino 2007).

The prevalence of this excessive crying varies according to the definition used, although, most often, it peaks during the second month of life with a prevalence of 1.5–11.9% (Reijneveld et al. 2001). The incidence of simple colic is estimated to be between 10% and 30% of infants at any one time (Clifford et al. 2002; Rosen et al. 2007).

However, about 5% of excessively crying infants do have a serious, underlying medical problem (Savino et al. 2005; Freedman et al. 2009), and there is evidence that older children presenting with migraine are more likely to have been babies who have suffered colic (Romanello et al. 2013). Because of this, babies with unresolved colicky symptoms which remain after attempts have been made to determine the cause and to manage the crying should undergo a complete medical assessment in order to exclude underlying medical conditions which require investigation and treatment (Savino and Tarasco 2010).

It has been suggested that a number of environmental factors, behavioural factors (psychological and social) and biological components (food hypersensitivity, allergy, gut microflora, bloating from trapped gas and dysmotility) can contribute to it (Gupta 2007).

A recent systematic review (Gordon et al. 2018) has identified various different potential causes of the colicky symptoms, ranging from trapped gas; to a problem with feeding such as under- or overfeeding or some inappropriate feed content; to allergy causing spasms and/or gut-lining damage and fermentation; and lactose intolerance causing fermentation and diarrhoea, and some other issue of unknown aetiology, but possibly microbial – so perhaps from some upset to the gut flora and fauna from receiving antibiotics, or even from being born by caesarean section.

Babies might take in air either through crying or during feeding. It is more common for bottlefed babies to take in air during feeding, but breastfed babies sometimes struggle when their mum has a fast let-down reflex or suboptimal positioning at the breast, as well. Additionally, missing the early feeding cues for either breastfed or bottlefed babies can mean that the baby gets upset and cries for feeds, which can increase the trapped gas.

Allergy and intolerance can cause fermentation in the stomach or gut, producing gas as a side effect. In the short term infants may have lactose intolerance after a gut insult such as gastroenteritis.

However the trapped gas is getting in there to begin with: knowing how to release the gas out of the stomach or to help with discomfort in the intestine is also key, and again, accessing expert and experienced infant feeding support for parents is likely to be effective (Welsh Government 2019).

There is growing evidence that the intestinal microbiota in colicky infants differ from those in non-colicky controls, since higher levels of anaerobic bacteria, such as coliform and *Escherichia coli*, and microaerophilic bacteria such as *Helicobacter pylori* (Ali 2012) have been reported in infants with colic, and a lower concentration of *Lactobacillus* (Savino et al. 2010).

In addition to probiotics (the 'healthy' bacteria), human milk naturally contains prebiotics (the food for the probiotic); these are indigestible oligosaccharides that could selectively enhance the proliferation of certain probiotic bacteria in the colon, especially *Bifidobacterium* species (Thomas and Greer 2010).

Some studies have failed to find a protective effect of breastfeeding on the development of colic in breastfed infants (Clifford et al. 2002); however, it is unclear if these studies compared exclusively breastfed-from-birth infants with exclusively artificially fed-from-birth infants, and so it is still not known whether any breastfeeding has some protective effect or whether any artificial feeding compromises the infant gut microbiome in some way.

However, in these times of large-scale deviation from the biological norms of vaginal birth, skin-to-skin contact after delivery and exclusive breastmilk feeding in the early months of life, it is easy to understand how an infant's microbiome may be altered from its intended formation by the absence of these events and the unintended gut colonisation of less favourable bacteria from the hospital, staff or feeding equipment. It is thought that the altered microbiota may be responsible for the colicky pain experienced by some infants and that prophylactically receiving probiotics might protect the infant from that colicky pain ever occurring, by steering the trajectory of microbial gut colonisation nearer to that which was intended (Indrio et al. 2014).

In addition to vaginal birth and early skin-to-skin contact, one of the most useful ways to manage microbial balance in the gut of an infant who is formula-fed is to ensure that the milk is being made up correctly, which reduces the risk of the gut being overrun by illness-causing bacteria. Obviously, a fully breastfed baby has a far greater chance of having a microbial balance which is appropriate for its environment, because the mother's own microbiome, accumulated over decades, will be shared with the baby in a reactive and responsive way via the milk.

Some studies have identified lactose intolerance as a possible causative factor in infantile colic (Kanabar et al. 2001), due to a relative lactase deficiency, which may mean either too much lactose (the milk sugar) to begin with, perhaps owing to the way the baby is breastfeeding, or too little of the enzyme lactase in the gut, meaning the milk sugar lactose (present in both breastmilk and infant formula, as in all animal milks) is not able to be digested. Poor absorption of the carbohydrate leads to fermentation of sugars in the gut, and an increase in the levels of hydrogen gas (Infante et al. 2011). The rapid production of hydrogen in the lower bowel bloats the colon, sometimes causing pain, while lactose and lactic acid in the colon cause an influx of water leading to further bloat (Indrio 2014). Although studies evaluating the degree of hydrogen in the breath of colicky infants have produced inconsistent results, increases in breath hydrogen levels have been reported (Moore et al. 1988; Hyams et al. 1989; Miller et al. 1990).

The most common allergen is cows' milk proteins in infant formula or even mothers' milk. Intact proteins from a mother's diet can sometimes cross over into the breast milk, provoking an allergic response and symptoms of colic in her infant. Consequently, a low-allergen maternal diet or hypoallergenic infant formula has been proposed as a form of treatment (Moore et al. 1988; Schach and Haight 2002; Hill and Hosking 2004) for the breastfed infant. Shannon (1921) first described the possibility of a relationship between infantile colic and allergens, and since then, a number of studies have evaluated the possible association between colic and food hypersensitivity (Lothe et al. 1982; Iacono et al. 1991; Hill et al. 1995; Heine 2013; Heine et al. 2014).

The evidence shows that about 25% of infants with moderate or severe symptoms have cows' milk, protein-dependent colic (Axelsson et al. 1986; Lindberg 1999; Hill and Hosking 2000), which improves after some days on a hypoallergenic diet (Lothe and Lindberg 1989; Gordon et al. 2018). For these infants, infantile colic could be the first manifestation of atopic disease, and for this reason, after practical feed management coming from someone who has taken a full history and observed a full feed, dietetic treatment should be one of the first therapeutic approaches (Gupta 2007; Savino and Tarasco 2010; Perry et al. 2011; Hall et al. 2012). Indeed, dietary changes are particularly indicated in cases of suspected intolerance to cows' milk proteins (for example, in infants with a positive family history; eczema or onset after the first month of life; or colic associated with other gastrointestinal symptoms, such as vomiting or diarrhoea) (Jakobsson and Lindberg 1983; Hill et al. 1995; Hill et al. 2005). If the baby is being formula-fed, then the infant will require a hypoallergenic or potentially an amino acid formula (Lucassen et al. 2000).

There is growing evidence that colic is 25% more prevalent in the babies of cigarette smokers and mothers who have used nicotine replacement in pregnancy and breastfeeding, suggesting that there is an intolerance of the nicotine itself (Milidou et al. 2012), which manifests in symptoms of colic.

Ensure the parents are well supported and can vent their frustrations somewhere safe. Promote stress management with parents – babies pick up on our anxiety and tension. If the parents are feeling overwhelmed, and all attempts to calm the child have failed, then sometimes it may be safer for them to put the child down in a safe place, and walk away into another room, to regroup their thoughts.

There is no clarity as to the extent these components contribute to the overall efficacy of symptom reduction strategies or to parental anxiety levels. Some interventions found to be effective in reducing parental anxiety have been found to be *ineffective* in reducing symptoms in the infant, such as in the 2010 study (McRury and Zolotor 2010) based on techniques found in a popular parenting book (Karp 2003). Given the clinical and methodological heterogeneity of studies on these interventions, the efficacy of these interventions in reducing infant colic remains inconclusive, at present.

Some parents will be keen to try over-the-counter pharmaceutical remedies. There are a variety of things sold to help with colicky symptoms, but they work in specific ways and address just one potential cause so won't work for everyone.

There is very little evidence that any of these treatments work, but the current guidelines suggest parents could trial them – for no longer than a week. There may be a placebo effect. Evidence of efficacy is not comprehensive (Garrison and Christakis 2000).

Infacol (simethicone) reduces the surface tension of bubbles of gas trapped in liquid, so they join together. Dentinox (dimethicone) is similar. Although systematic reviews have failed to provide evidence of its efficacy in reducing colicky symptoms by reducing trapped gas in the liquid of the stomach, simethicone is still often used (Metcalf et al. 1994).

Lactase drops (Colief, Co-Lactase and LactAid) help break down lactose in the milk if the body has a lactase shortage or the milk has too much lactose for the body to handle – it cannot work to reduce stomach symptoms, because the effects of too much lactose or not enough of the enzyme lactase are felt from the intestine onwards.

Gripe water has different ingredients depending on the brand, but the UK's most sold brand contains dill oil which claims to 'warm and relax the tummy, breaking down trapped air bubbles' and sodium hydrogen carbonate which they claim 'neutralises acid in the baby's tummy'. These are non-evidenced claims: 5 mL of drinkable liquid does not contain enough to change the temperature or pH of the stomach substantially. Additionally, sodium bicarbonate works on the hydrochloric acid in the stomach, forming a combination of sodium chloride, carbon dioxide and water – so gripe water will actually *cause* the formation of gas in the stomach.

It's thought that the action of the dill may actually be as an oligosaccharide (complex carbohydrate) which feeds the friendly bacteria, and the reason gripe water seems to work is that it tastes nice to the baby so the infant is simply happier. Of course, when many of us were babies, gripe water contained alcohol!

Recently some 'probiotic' products have started to be marketed to parents, to be given directly to baby; as discussed above, there is an argument for supplementing the microbiome of a baby whose microbiome has been compromised by its method of birth, illness of the mother, smoking in the home, formula feeding or some other factor. However, to do that successfully, we would need to know what was missing from the microbiome.

Many studies have been conducted (Savino 2007; Savino and Tarasco 2010; Dupont et al. 2010; Szajewski et al. 2013) into the use of oral probiotics to manage infantile colic, and a Cochrane systematic review of the currently available evidence has recently been completed examining the effects of probiotics for preventing infantile colic (Ong et al. 2019). However the studies have not proven which strains are most likely to be effective or indeed safe in management of symptoms.

Some parents choose to try herbal or dietary strategies such as fennel or peppermint tea. Some complementary and alternative medicines such as fennel extract (Harb et al. 2016) and chamomile (Perry et al. 2011) have been trialled but do not have demonstrable efficacy.

Gastro-oesophageal reflux

Gastro-oesophageal reflux (GOR) is the normal physiological regurgitation of an infant's milk up from the stomach into the oesophagus, and sometimes up and out of the mouth, ranging from a 'swallowing down', through small amounts of posset, right the way up to projectile regurgitation of what seems like a full feed (NICE 2015). Thinking about it logically, the physical immaturity of the gastro-oesophageal sphincter, combined with the horizontal position of babies, provides a pressure upon the sphincter which may simply allow stomach contents to be pushed up – or sideways – into the oesophagus, much as if one carried a plastic container of home-made soup on its side in one's bag to work. This regurgitation is very common, and usually presents no problem for the child, merely a laundry issue for the parents! However, of course, in some cases, regurgitation can lead to problems with weight gain and some distress for the infant, either from the force of the regurgitation or from the passage of stomach acid up into the oesophagus and resultant damage to its lining.

Because their bodies are new and immature, and because we keep lying them down, it's very normal for babies to experience this physiological reflux – some GOR occurs in most babies. An estimated 40–50% of babies under 3 months regurgitate their feed at least once a day (Craig et al. 2004) and it is particularly common in preterm infants, younger babies and those with neurodevelopmental disorders or hernias – even if repaired (Tidy et al. 2018). Incidence peaks around 4 months.

Research is consistent that frequency of regurgitation declines over the first 6 months and dramatically after 12 months (Szajewski et al. 2013). This interestingly corresponds with the time when babies can sit and stand, therefore their stomach is less restricted, precipitating posseting.

Sometimes the cause of both colic and reflux might be the same: trapped gas caused by a problem with feed management, or some fermentation in the gut from an overload of lactose because the baby is not well attached at the breast, or an allergy to something in the milk, such as (most commonly) cows' milk protein, soy protein or other proteins such as from fish, egg or wheat. Occasionally the reaction is to something more unusual, but usually in conjunction with something more common, such as a cows' milk protein allergy rather than a stand-alone unusual reaction. Clearly the route if an allergy via mum's milk is a genuine possibility (many mums have read about cows' milk protein allergy on the internet, but it actually isn't the first thing to consider) is to cut cows' milk protein from the maternal diet.

GOR is distinct from GORD, which is gastro-oesophageal reflux disease. If symptoms of GOR are associated with respiratory disorders or suspected oesophagitis, it is termed GORD. Here again diagnosis is made on clinical symptoms and NICE (2015) offers a cluster of symptoms to guide prescribing.

NICE guidance

Signs which may suggest a diagnosis of GORD:

- The baby is not gaining weight.
- The baby vomits frequently and forcefully.
- The baby spits up green or yellow fluid.
- The baby spits up a liquid which looks like coffee grounds.
- The baby repeatedly refuses feeds.
- The baby has blood in the bowel motions.

NICE (2015) reports that overfeeding is a common cause in artificially fed infants who may benefit from smaller, more frequent bottlefeeds. However it also suggests a common scenario in which infants with frequent regurgitation are taken to see the GP; a prescription may be offered to alleviate parents' concerns that the regurgitation is abnormal. The medication may be unnecessary if the infant is otherwise well, and is gaining weight. Advice and reassurance that GOR is normal and will resolve in time are preferable.

They suggest that GOR is not routinely investigated or treated if an infant or child without overt regurgitation presents with only one of the following:

- unexplained feeding difficulties;
- distressed behaviour;
- faltering growth;
- chronic cough;
- hoarseness;
- a single episode of pneumonia.

In formula-fed infants with frequent regurgitation associated with marked distress (potentially GORD), the following stepped-care approach is recommended:

- review the feeding history, then
- reduce the feed volumes only if excessive for the infant's weight, then offer a trial of smaller, more frequent feeds (while maintaining an appropriate total daily amount of milk) unless the feeds are already small and frequent, then offer a trial of thickened formula (recommendation 1.2.3).

Although there is also evidence that thickened feeds are not effective in reducing overall reflux, NICE suggests that if the stepped-care approach is unsuccessful, stop the thickened formula and offer alginate therapy (for example, Gaviscon Infant sachets, or Carobel) for a trial period of 1–2 weeks. If the alginate therapy is successful continue with it but try stopping it at intervals to see if the infant has recovered. The sachets of alginate should be dissolved in water or expressed breastmilk, as described below. However, alginates are constipating as they thicken the gastric contents. This may cause further distress to the baby and parents and anecdotally can lead to prescription of bulk-forming laxatives in addition to the alginate.

In breast-fed infants with frequent regurgitation associated with marked distress, NICE guidance is to ensure that a person with appropriate expertise and training carries out a breastfeeding assessment. If the frequent regurgitation associated with marked distress continues, despite a breastfeeding assessment and appropriate breastfeeding management changes, consider alginate therapy for a trial period of 1–2 weeks. If the alginate therapy is successful continue with it but try stopping it at intervals to see if the infant has recovered.

Silent reflux is described as reflux where the regurgitation is swallowed rather than being regurgitated: babies may cry and show signs of distress but not posset. Symptoms may otherwise be identical to GOR, and present as 'colic'.

With GOR, medication is unnecessary. However, parents may wish to try remedies to relieve symptoms of excessive crying and posseting in their babies. Medication should not be commenced without prior referral to an expert in breastfeeding to optimise attachment.

Acid-suppressing drugs, such as proton pump inhibitors (PPIs) or H2 receptor antagonists (H2RAs), should not be used to treat overt regurgitation occurring as an isolated symptom in infants and children.

Some studies looking at the effectiveness of Gaviscon and of the antiemetic metoclopramide in treating the symptoms of GOR have found that they decreased neither frequency nor duration of GOR; however the study sizes are small and the results inconsistent.

From a GP cost perspective ranitidine is the cheapest option, then omeprazole tablets (to be constituted by parents), and then Gaviscon, which is the most expensive with the sachets costing roughly £1 per day. Pre-made omeprazole suspension is considerably more expensive.

Colic and reflux are sometimes symptoms of allergy

There is some good evidence that reflux may be a symptom of cows' milk allergy or intolerance, so it is worth keeping a food and symptom diary.

The most common allergen in infants is cows' milk proteins in infant formula or even mothers' milk. Where there are allergies there are often other allergies, often egg and fish (ingredients in some types of infant formula) and soy, wheat and nuts.

Intact proteins from a mother's diet can sometimes cross over into the breast milk, provoking an allergic response and regurgitation in her infant. Consequently, a low-allergen maternal diet or hypoallergenic infant formula has been proposed as a form of treatment (Caffarelli et al. 2010). A number of studies have evaluated the possible association between reflux and food hypersensitivity (Vandenplas and Hauser 2015).

The evidence shows that about 25% of infants with moderate or severe symptoms have cows' milk, protein-triggered reflux, which improves after some days on a hypoallergenic diet. For these infants, the regurgitation could be the first manifestation of atopic disease, and for this reason, dietetic treatment should be one of the first therapeutic approaches. Indeed, dietary changes are particularly indicated in cases of suspected intolerance to cows' milk proteins (for example, in infants with a positive family history; eczema or onset after the first month of life; or indeed reflux).

A promising area of research within allergy is the role of epigenetics, which describes the modification of substances within the DNA strand that regulate gene expression (DeVries and Vercelli 2015).

One of the main mechanisms by which genes can be activated or silenced is the process of adding a substance called a methyl group to the DNA strand. DNA methylation modifies a particular gene and fixes it in the 'off' position. DNA methylation is essential for healthy growth and development and enables the suppression of pathogenic or faulty genes which might otherwise cause harm. Abnormal methylation silences genes which are supposed to be suppressed – such as cancer and allergy.

Breast milk has been shown to influence and optimise DNA methylation (Hartwig et al. 2017) whereas formula milk causes abnormal methylation (because it contains cow DNA, not human DNA). This means that formula milk exposure can cause the allergy suppression gene to be switched 'off' – so that the infant becomes more susceptible to allergy. Changes to the DNA code are passed to future generations, meaning that even with optimal feeding and care practices the infant may exhibit the effects of suboptimal gene expression caused by infant care and feeding practices in the generations before.

Genes can be expressed to a greater or lesser extent. In fact, genetic expression is a bit like a dimmer switch, rather than a simple on/off switch. The more faulty the methylation mechanism, the more the switch is turned 'off' for allergic suppression (meaning the infant experiences more symptoms of allergy).

At least 24% of all disease is modifiable or affected by nutrition, stress and toxins (Prüss-Üstün and Corvalán 2006).

The immune system is most vulnerable in the first 1,000 days after conception, which makes pregnancy and the first 2 years of a child's life the most critical in terms of nutrition to support lifelong health. The infant's gut is immature, and 'leaky' in the first few months after birth. It is designed to be protected with the immunoglobulins in breastmilk (Hanson and Söderström 1981).

Caring for a baby with reflux is difficult, exhausting and confusing. It may be isolating as the mother may be concerned about the baby posseting when outside the family home. Does she have enough changes of clothes for herself and the baby? What will other people say? What if the regurgitated milk goes on to someone or something else? The mother may feel a loss in confidence as well as exhaustion. Being told that her baby's symptoms are normal may be somewhat reassuring, but may also leave her feeling helpless and belittled. Listening to the parents' concerns, and believing them, before seeking to find a solution, is a vital first step.

Most cases of reflux clear up over time, but simple changes can help reduce symptoms:

- Feed more frequently and respond at the baby's first cues that s/he is hungry: crying is a late sign of hunger and increases air swallowing, making regurgitation of feeds more likely.
- Ensure that baby's feeding position and style, whether breast or bottle, does not result in the baby swallowing air with its milk.
- Keep the baby upright after feeds over the shoulder, ideally for at least 30 minutes. Do not put the baby down in a car seat or bouncy chair where the baby slumps. Try not to jiggle or move the baby too much as the feed settles.
- Take time to wind baby in an upright position with the baby's head supported by the carer's hand – be prepared with a muslin cloth over the shoulder and a bib on the baby to protect clothing (and reduce washing!).
- When putting the baby down to sleep flat on the back, the whole of one end of the crib can be raised so that the crib mattress is flat but sloping down from head end to foot end to raise the head or upper body of the baby only. However avoid the use of pillows or wedges.
- Ensure that breastfeeding management has been optimised to ensure the baby has access to all the milk and that the mother's breasts are well drained after a breast-feed; ensure an appropriately qualified individual is involved in the dyad's care.

References

Ali A (2012) *Helicobacter pylori* and infantile colic. *Arch Pediatr Adolesc Med* 166(7):648–50.

Axelsson I, Jakobsson I, Lindberg T, Benediktsson B (1986) Bovine beta-lactoglobulin in the human milk. A longitudinal study during the whole lactation period. *Acta Paediatr Scand* 75(5):702–7.

Caffarelli C, Baldi F, Bendandi B, Calzone L, Pasquinelli P (2010) Cow's milk protein allergy in children: a practical guide. *Ital J Pediatr* 15(36):5.

Clifford T, Campbell M, Speechley K, Gorodzinski F (2002) Infant colic: empirical evidence of the absence of an association with source of early infant nutrition. *Arch Pediatr Adolesc Med* 156(11):1123–8.

Craig W, Hanlon-Dearman E, Sinclair C, Taback S, Moffatt M (2004) Metoclopramide, thickened feedings, and positioning for gastro-oesophageal reflux in children under two years. *Cochrane Library*, p. 4.

DeVries A, Vercelli D (2015) Epigenetics in allergic diseases. *Pediatrics* 27(6):719–23.

Dupont C, Rivero M, Grillon C, Belaroussi N, Kalindjian A, Marin V (2010) Alpha-lactalbumin-enriched and probiotic-supplemented infant formula in infants with colic: growth and gastro-intestinal tolerance. *Eur J Clin Nutr* 64(7):765–7.

Freedman S, Al-Harthy N, Thull-Freedman J (2009) The crying infant: diagnostic testing and frequency of serious underlying disease. *Pediatrics* 123(3):841–8.

Garrison M, Christakis D (2000) A systematic review of treatments for infant colic. *Pediatrics* 106(1 pt 2):184–90.

Gordon M, Biagioli E, Lingua C, Moja L, Banks S, Savino F (2018) Dietary modifications for infantile colic. *Cochrane Library*.

Gupta S (2007) Update on infantile colic and management options. *Investig Drugs* 8(11):921–6.

Hall B, Chesters J, Robinson A (2012) Infantile colic: a systematic review of medical and conventional therapies. *J Paediatr Child Health* 48(2):128–37.

Hanson L, Söderström T (1981) Human milk: defense against infection. *Prog Clin Biol Res* 61:147–59.

Harb T, Matsuyama M, David M, Hill R (2016) Infant colic – what works: a systematic review of interventions for breast-fed infants. *J Pediatr Gastroenterol Nutr* 62(5):668–86.

Hartwig F, Loreto de Mola C, Davies M, Victora C, Relton C (2017) Breastfeeding effects on DNA methylation in the offspring: a systematic literature review. *PloS One* 12(3):e0173070.

Heine R (2013) Cow's-milk allergy and lactose malabsorption in infants with colic. *J Paediatr Gastroenterol Nutr* 57(Suppl 1):S25–7.

Heine R, Hill D, Hoskin C (2014) Infantile colic and food allergy. In: *Food Allergy: Adverse Reactions to Foods and Food Additives*, 5th ed. Chichester: John Wiley, pp. 171–81.

Hill D, Hosking C (2000) Infantile colic and food hypersensitivity. *J Pediatr Gastroenterol Nutr* 30:S67–76.

Hill D, Hudson I, Sheffield L, Shelton M, Menahem S, Hosking C (1995) A low allergen diet is a significant intervention in infantile colic: results of a community-based study. *J Allergy Clin Immunol* 96(6):886–92.

Hill D, Hosking C, Roy N, Carlin J, Francis D, Brown J (2004) Colic in breast fed infants is due to hypersensitivity to dietary proteins excreted in breast milk. *J Allergy Clin Immunol* 113(2)(Suppl):S338.

Hill D, Roy N, Heine R, Hosking C, Francis D, Brown J (2005) Effect of a low-allergen maternal diet on colic among breastfed infants: a randomized, controlled trial. *Pediatrics* 116(5):e709–15.

Hyams J, Geertsma M, Etienne N, Treem W (1989) Colonic hydrogen production in infants with colic. *J Pediatr* 115(4):592–4.

Iacono G, Carroccio A, Montalto G, Cavataio F, Bragion E, Lorello D (1991) Severe infantile colic and food intolerance: a long-term prospective study. *J Pediatr Gastroenterol Nutr* 12(3):332–5.

Indrio F, Di Mauro A, Riezzo G, Civardi E, Intini C, Corvaglia L (2014) Prophylactic use of a probiotic in the prevention of colic, regurgitation, and functional constipation: a randomized clinical trial. *JAMA Pediatr* 168(3):228–33.

Infante D, Segarra O, Luyer B (2011) Dietary treatment of colic caused by excess gas in infants: biochemical evidence. *World J Gastroenterol* 17(16):2104–8.

Jakobsson I, Lindberg T (1983) Cow's milk proteins cause infantile colic in breast-fed infants: a double-blind crossover study. *Pediatrics* 71(2):268–713.

Kanabar D, Randhawa M, Clayton P (2001) Improvement of symptoms in infant colic following reduction of lactose load with lactase. *J Hum Nutr Dietet* 14(5):359–63.

Karp H (2003) *The Happiest Baby on the Block*. New York: Bantam.

Koppen I, Nurko S, Saps M, Di Lorenzo C, Benninga M (2017) The pediatric Rome IV criteria: what's new? *Gastroenterol Hepatol* 11(3):193–201.

Lindberg T (1999) Infantile colic and small intestinal function: a nutritional problem? *Acta Paediatr* 88(430):58–60.

Lothe L, Lindberg T (1989) Cow's milk whey protein elicits symptoms of infantile colic in colicky formula-fed infants: a double-blind crossover study. *Pediatrics* 83(2):262–6.

Lothe T, Lindberg T, Jakobsson I (1982) Cow's milk formula as a cause of infantile colic: a double-blind study. *Pediatrics* 70(1):7–10.

Lucas A, St James-Roberts I (1998) Crying, fussing and colic behaviour in breast- and bottle-fed infants. *Early Hum Dev* 53(1):9–18.

Lucassen P, Assendelft W, Gubbels J, Eijk J, Douwes A (2000) Infantile colic: crying time reduction with a whey hydrolysate: a dle-blind, randomized, placebo-controlled trial. *Pediatrics* 106(6):1349–54.

McRury J, Zolotor A (2010) A randomized, controlled trial of a behavioral intervention to reduce crying among infants. J Am Board Fam Med 23(3):315–22.

Metcalf T, Irons T, Sher L, Young P (1994) Simethicone in the treatment of infant colic: a randomized, placebo-controlled, multicenter trial. *Pediatrics* 94(1):29–34.

Milidou I, Henriksen T, Jensen M, Olsen J, Søndergaard C (2012) Nicotine replacement therapy during pregnancy and infantile colic in the offspring. *Pediatrics* 129(3):e652–8.

Miller J, McVeagh P, Fleet G, Petocz P, Brand J (1990) Effect of yeast lactase enzyme on "colic" in infants fed human milk. *J Pediatr* 117(2):261–3.

Moore D, Robb T, Davidson G (1988) Breath hydrogen response to milk containing lactose in colicky and noncolicky infants. *J Pediatr* 113(6):979–84.

NICE (2015) *Gastro-oesophageal Reflux Disease in Children and Young People: Diagnosis and Management.* National Institute for Health & Clinical Excellence. www.nice.org.uk/ guidance/ng1

Ong T, Gordon M, Banks S, Thomas M, Akobeng A (2019) Probiotics to prevent infantile colic. *Cochrane Library*.

Perry R, Hunt K, Ernst E (2011) Nutritional supplements and other complementary medicines for infantile colic: a systematic review. *Pediatrics* 127(4):720–33.

Prüss-Üstün A, Corvalán C (2006) Preventing disease through healthy environments: Towards an estimate of the environmental burden of disease. World Health Organization. https://apps. who.int/iris/handle/10665/43457

Reijneveld S, Brugman E, Hirasing R (2001) Excessive infant crying: the impact of varying definitions. *Pediatrics* 108(4):893–7.

Romanello S, Spiri D, Marcuzzi E, Zanin A, Boizeau P, Riviere S (2013) Association between childhood migraine and history of infantile colic. *JAMA* 309(15):1607–12.

Rosen L, Bukutu C, Le C, Shamseer L, Vohrer S (2007) Complementary, holistic, and integrative medicine: colic. *Pediatr Rev* 28(10):381–5.

Savino F (2007) Focus on infantile colic. *Acta Paediatr* 96(9):1259–64.

Savino F, Tarasco V (2010) New treatments for infant colic. *Pediatrics* 22(6): 791–7.

Savino F, Castagno E, Bretto R, Brondello C, Palumeri E, Oggero R (2005) A prospective 10-year study on children who had severe infantile colic. *Acta Paediatr Suppl* 94(449):129–32.

Savino F, Pelle E, Palumeri E, Oggero R, Miniero R (2007) *Lactobacillus reuteri* (American type culture collection strain 55730) versus simethicone in the treatment of infantile colic: a prospective randomized study. *Pediatrics* 119(1):e124–30.

Savino F, Cordisco L, Tarasco V, Palumeri E, Calabrese R, Oggero R (2010) *Lactobacillus reuteri* DSM 17938 in infantile colic: a randomized, double-blind, placebo-controlled trial. *Pediatrics* 1(3):e526–33.

Schach B, Haight M (2002) Colic and food allergy in the breastfed infant: is it possible for an exclusively breastfed infant to suffer from food allergy? *J Hum Lactat* 18(1):50–2.

Shannon WR (1921) Colic in breast-fed infants as a result of sensitization to foods in the mother's diet. Arch Paediatr 38:756–61.

Szajewski H, Gyrczuk E, Horvath A (2013) *Lactobacillus reuteri* DSM 17938 for the management of infantile colic in breastfed infants: a randomized, double-blind, placebo-controlled trial. *J Pediatr* 162(2):257–62.

Thomas D, Greer F (2010) Probiotics and prebiotics in pediatrics. *Pediatrics* 126(6):1217–31.

Tidy DC (2018) Childhood Gastro-oesophageal Reflux. Patient information. https://patient. info/doctor/gastro-oesophageal-reflux-disease

Vandenplas Y, Hauser B (2015) An updated review in gastro-oesophageal reflux. *Pediatrics* 9(12):1511–21.

Welsh Government (2018) A Review of Breastfeeding support and practices in the Maternity and Early Years settings in Wales.. https://gov.wales/sites/default/files/publications/2019-03/ a-review-of-breastfeeding-support-and-practices-in-the-maternity-and-early-years-settings- in-wales.pdf

Wessel M, Cobb J, Jackson E, Harris G, Detwiler A (1954) Paroxysmal fussing in infancy, sometimes called colic. *Pediatrics* 14(5):421–35.

13 Why provide donor human milk?

Natalie Shenker

Having twin girls born prematurely brought equal measures of joy and terror. The start was particularly rough and emotionally difficult, as I wasn't able to see the babies myself until I was medically more stable. I'd had a difficult pregnancy, and was managing hypertension and gestational diabetes when I was diagnosed with pre-eclampsia. My twins were born by emergency C-section at 33 weeks, and I don't remember much of the first few hours after they were born. I'd desperately wanted to breastfeed them. Having donor milk available lifted such a huge weight from me. Sitting in the obstetric close observation unit, desperately trying to express my own milk, fluid restricted due to dangerously low sodium levels and unable to visit my babies was horrendous. When the donor milk arrived, I sobbed with relief and gratitude. Donor milk meant that I could be sure they would be getting the benefit of the rich and varied composition of breastmilk whilst protecting their tiny and immature gut. I guess what I'm saying is that donor milk made the difference between despair and hope. It gave me space to breathe and heal.

Within a day their sugars were stable, two days later, they had their lines out, two days after that they were out of incubators and on to warming cots – a combination of my milk and donor human milk in action. It was estimated we wouldn't be home until after their term date, but we came home three weeks early. Things have been and remain intense, but we are settling into our lives as parents.

There's no substitute for human milk – the impact it has can be seen in our babies. It staggers us that a national logistics system for donor milk similar to the national blood bank has never existed. Every parent and child should have access to the milk they need in a way that supports both mothers and children, no matter where they are or what their circumstances.

(Jo, mum to premature twins)

For babies who are unable to receive their mother's own milk, donor human milk (DHM) can play an important role in protecting their health and supporting their development. When used in the context of early lactation support by trained neonatal unit staff, the availability of DHM can markedly increase maternal breastfeeding rates (Kantorowska et al. 2016). Dr Camilla Kingdon, who led the establishment of the human milk bank (HMB) at St Thomas's Hospital in London in the early 2000s, explained that maternal breastfeeding rates on discharge went from 35% to over 70% within the first 2 years of implementation (C. Kingdon, personal communication).

Over 15 years later, the cultural change in attitudes towards human milk means the unit now has discharge rates of 90–95% of any breastfeeding, which includes babies who have had long stays on the neonatal intensive care unit (NICU).

Many doctors avoid using DHM precisely for the reason that it may make mothers less motivated to spend large amounts of time expressing milk for their babies. And it is true that when DHM is introduced to neonatal units, rates of maternal own milk (MOM) feeding can go down (Parker et al. 2019). The critical point is that DHM used in isolation can absolutely demotivate mothers to persevere with establishing their own supply. Clues are also apparent from small qualitative studies in other countries. When babies are born preterm or sick, maternal stress levels are unavoidably high. The mother may be ill herself, or physically separated, sometimes in a different part of a hospital, or another hospital altogether. Mothers may feel under intense pressure to produce milk – breastmilk is often described to parents as acting like a medicine, nurturing development, preventing pathogen invasion through oligosaccharide binding to pathogens (Bode 2012; Lin et al. 2017; Triantis et al. 2018), dysbiosis and the promotion of gut maturity (Groer 2015) and driving brain development (Blesa et al. 2019). From qualitative interviews, mothers who are unable to provide full feeds to their babies are more likely to perceive their bodies as having 'failed' if formula is used, while DHM is seen as a bridge to establishing a full supply (Kair et al. 2015; Kair and Flaherman 2017).

In November 2017, PATH, a global non-governmental organisation that drives healthcare improvements globally using technology, published a report in collaboration with the World Health Organization (WHO) and UNICEF that reiterated previous recommendations that donor milk was the best supplement to maternal milk for very low-birthweight babies. This is in line with guidance from the American Association of Pediatrics (https://pediatrics.aappublications.org/content/139/1/e20163440), and the European Society for Pediatric Gastroenterology, Hepatology and Nutrition (Arslanoglu et al. 2013). HMB numbers are increasing worldwide, critically in resource-poor countries (DeMarchis et al. 2016) where low-cost technological solutions are being rapidly developed to assist with donor screening and milk processing. Many of these tools can also enhance the cost-effectiveness of milk banking in developed-world countries. The last 20 years have seen a marked growth in the number of HMBs and the use of DHM. Currently, over 600 HMBs exist in 60 countries compared with fewer than 500 in 50 countries 5 years ago. Existing HMBs have also grown in size to provide more DHM to neonatal units (NNUs). The result is a widespread increase in the number of infants receiving DHM globally. It is also common for mothers of NNU infants to be recruited as milk donors.

Historically, women have donated their milk through wet nursing or sharing for millennia. This was semi-formalised over the last century with the advent of largely hospital-based milk banks, which brought in safety measures such as pasteurisation and microbiological screening. During the 1960s and 1970s in the UK, milk sharing was common on postnatal units, either semi-formally with pasteurisation or some form of flash heat treatment ('containers put in pans of boiling water') or simply with mothers with a good milk supply asked to express milk for another mother's baby, or even feed directly at the breast. The awareness that HIV could be transmitted through breastmilk during the 1980s effectively stopped all except the units that had access to pasteurisers, and trained staff who could operate them. By 1991, only six milk banks were left in the UK. The reason that these six survived was largely the prevention of necrotising enterocolitis (NEC), and the passionate defence of milk banks by individual clinicians. Why were there not more clinical advocates at that stage? Largely because infant formula companies, reeling from the public reaction to press exposure of their activities in the developing world during the 1970s and 1980s, had diversified their infant feeding portfolio into specialised medical formulas – and they started with preterm formula. Essentially, it was the same product – powdered cows' milk with variations in the supplementation of vitamins and minerals – but repackaged and marketed as essential for the health of premature and very sick babies. And these products were not marketed at parents, but at doctors. Why bother rebuilding a national milk bank service infrastructure, with all of the inherent costs, when a suitable alternative that costs very little is available?

The problem is, the human neonatal gut is not expecting to be fed with cows' milk protein, which can cause an array of reactions (including inflammation and immune system blunting).

Since the 1990s, when milk bank services were limited, donor milk has been almost exclusively rationed to feed extremely preterm babies, whose own mothers cannot provide enough of their own milk. Infants are usually fed on average for just 5 days. Mothers whose babies have received donor milk, along with appropriate support and information, are significantly more likely to go on to establish breastfeeding themselves. Human milk for sick babies acts like a medicine – the hundreds of bioactive components within milk act to promote gut development, a healthy microbiome, optimal brain development and a mature immune system. Even after freezing and heat treatment (pasteurisation), which donor milk undergoes to ensure safety, the majority of these components are intact and functional (Groer et al. 2014; Coscia et al. 2015; Peila et al. 2016). The overwhelming majority of these components are not found in infant formula, or are biochemically different and therefore will have different bioactivities *in vivo* (e.g. bovine vs. human lactoferrin).

The increased availability and use of donor milk are part of a cultural shift that recognises recent advances in human milk science and its impact on the developing, immature gut. Infants supplemented with formula have worsened outcomes in terms of both short- and long-term health. The available evidence shows utility for the use of donor milk in the following areas:

1. improved rates of maternal breastfeeding, when used in the context of lactation support and staff training (Kantorowska et al. 2016; Wilson et al. 2018).
2. species-specific milk leads to ease of digestion with minimal metabolic stress, which contributes to shortened duration to achieving full feeds, and reduced durations of hospital stay (Renfrew et al. 2009; Chowning et al. 2016), in the region of one night of NICU saved if all low-birthweight babies had access to donor milk. A night on the NICU in the UK ranges from £1200 to £2000. Parents report babies fed with human milk appear to have less discomfort, which alleviates some of their own stress;
3. potentially improved brain (Blesa et al. 2019) and cardiac development (Lewandowski 2016) and metabolic function (de Rooy and Hawdon 2002), largely mediated through the presence of essential fatty acids (arachidonic acid, docosahexanoic acid) that are unaffected by pasteurisation;
4. reduced rates and severity of complications of prematurity, including bronchopulmonary dysplasia (Villamor-Martínez et al. 2018) and retinopathy of prematurity (Zhou et al. 2015);

5. NEC: the principal driver for the maintenance of even limited donor milk provision to the most preterm babies has yielded studies that have been compiled into three meta-analyses to date, in 2007, 2014 and 2018. All three have shown an increase in the rates and severity of NEC, with high mortality rates particularly in surgical cases (Allin et al. 2017; Allin et al. 2018), leaving sufferers with long-term additional health needs (Boyd et al. 2007; Quigley and McGuire 2014; Niño et al. 2016; Quigley et al. 2018). These findings were supported by the largest randomised controlled trial to date in very low-birthweight babies, showing a near fourfold reduction in the relative risk of NEC with exclusive human milk feeds (O'Connor et al. 2016), although the trial was not powered to generate conclusions about NEC.

Debates around donor milk have largely revolved around cost, availability, efficacy for NEC and the lack of a firm evidence base to make any substantial decisions about funding a national service (BAPM 2016). NEC is a devastating and poorly understood condition, which kills more babies each year than leukaemia. Several factors contribute to an increased risk of a baby developing NEC, and some babies will develop NEC even when fed with just their mother's milk, or with donor milk as a supplement (Boyd et al. 2007; Quigley and McGuire 2014; Quigley et al. 2018). But when taking into consideration whole populations, feeding premature and sick babies with solely human milk seems to help reduce risk. It should be emphasised that NEC is not solely a disease of prematurity – 7% of surgically treated NEC during a year-long UK audit of care were in babies born >37 weeks' gestation (Allin et al. 2017).

Clinicians sometimes argue that the resources spent on milk banking services could be favourably redirected into supporting mothers to establish their supply in the NICU. However, as shown in Figure 13.1, the two are not separate entities, but

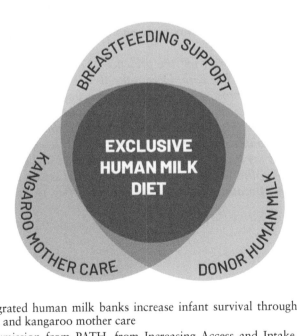

Figure 13.1 Integrated human milk banks increase infant survival through access to human milk and kangaroo mother care

Source: With permission from PATH, from Increasing Access and Intake of Human Milk: www.path.org/programs/maternal-newborn-child-health-and-nutrition/strengthening-human-milk-banking-resource-toolkit/.

mutual parts of a whole. There is a more compelling reason for DHM to be available, and that is the impact on parents of inequitable access. If a baby dies of NEC, and neither maternal nor DHM was available so formula had been used, those parents will never know whether DHM would have made a difference. Their anger is a pain that stays with them forever. The continuing debates around the provision of DHM arise because of the unsatisfactory or non-existent trial data that currently exist, which have impeded investment in services (BAPM 2016). How often could this be said for other interventions widely used in neonatology and paediatrics? Some parents may not choose DHM for their babies, but unavailability can leave an uncertainty that can last a lifetime if a baby dies.

Moreover, the nature of research into infant feeding is fundamentally changing with the first reporting of results from prospective studies that have recorded detailed day-by-day feeding information from large numbers of families. A prospective study has recently shown evidence of a subtly altered microbiome in babies fed with only small volumes of infant formula in hospital in an otherwise solely breastfed babies (Forbes et al. 2018), and that these babies are at a higher risk of being overweight at 1 year (Forbes et al. 2018; Moossavi and Azad 2019); if this result is corroborated by further studies, we may need to start thinking differently about using formula for supplementation in both sick and healthy babies.

> For two days my scant production was supplemented with donor milk. In their first days the feeding tube went into their mouths, for their nostrils were too little even for the tiniest of lines. A syringe was screwed on to the top of the tube, the plunger depressed, the whole 'feed' over in moments – 0.5 mL is about five drops, less than you would feed a day-old kitten. But those scant droplets were keeping my daughters alive. I stood by, feeling useless, guilty, grateful. I had failed to keep them safe inside my body and now I was failing to provide the scant nourishment they needed.
>
> But somewhere out there I felt the presence of another mother – and I felt supported, nurtured by her care. Here, take this. I have, you need. I felt so close to her I could almost see her face. She was anonymous, yet there were things I knew about her: she had a new baby. Without doubt, she had her own worries. Yet her generosity made possible the miracles that were my daughters. She offered up her antibodies to newborns in a state of terrifying immune compromise. She held my hand and we shielded the babies as best we could from necrotising enterocolitis (death of the bowel) and from sepsis, from deadly bacteria and viruses. Because of her, I was granted space to heal, to catch up, to learn.
>
> (Francesca Segal from Segal 2019, with permission)

Who are the donors?

Milk is donated altruistically by mothers who express milk that is surplus to their own baby's requirements. This might be because they are at home with a healthy baby and have an oversupply or are returning to work and pumping extra feeds to maintain their supply. It might be because their baby refuses to feed any other way than at the breast, or an oversupply has been stimulated by early pumping, or that they have simply added an extra pumping session to their daily routine in order to help other babies. Between 25% and 30% of milk donors donate their milk during or after a stay in hospital with a sick baby. In these cases, large excess volumes of frozen milk can build up very quickly. Sadly, some babies do not survive, and mothers can be supported to donate their milk in memory of their child. In this context, being able to donate milk can provide solace, a feeling that some good could come by helping other families at the most difficult of times (Kennedy et al. 2017). Sadly, many milk banks do not currently accept milk from bereaved donors, mainly as a result of a lack of trained staff able to support mothers. It is an area that requires much more investment in understanding options after baby loss, developing training and communication strategies in hospitals and the community, and upskilling and enhancing milk bank teams to provide this vital service.

Milk banks assume donated milk will be used to feed 23-week gestation premature babies. Safety is at the heart of everything done. Donors are supported to minimise the risk of bacterial contamination of the milk through advice with hand washing, pump sterilisation or hand-expressing techniques, storage (e.g. milk should be placed in the fridge as soon as possible and frozen to <–18°C within 24 hours (NICE 2010)). Other potential or theoretical risks are minimised through the completion of interviews and questionnaires that form a picture of a donor's health, health of the baby, medication use and any lifestyles that may impact the provision of milk to the most fragile babies. Some milk banks will also ask about diet, as the fats in particular vary according to maternal diet (Figure 13.2). Donors will then undergo blood tests for HIV-1 and 2,

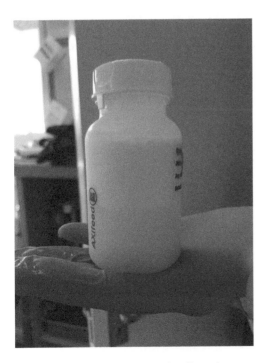

Figure 13.2 Defrosted donated milk to the Hearts Milk Bank showing separation. Fats rise and fatty components in this sample make up more than 50% by volume. The donor regularly ate oily fish

hepatitis B and C, syphilis and human T-lymphocytic virus (HTLV), which is endemic in southeast Asia and causes a form of leukaemia in approximately 1 in 20 carriers. All are transmissible through breastfeeding, but all are destroyed by pasteurisation. Other viruses, such as cytomegalovirus, are quickly destroyed by heat treatment, and are not part of the screening process. In some countries, such as Norway and parts of Germany, unpasteurised DHM is given to NICU babies and milk is only pasteurised if donors test positive for cytomegalovirus.

What happens to the milk?

DHM undergoes multiple processes on its journey, including freezing, thawing and heat treatment, as shown in Figure 13.3. Pasteurisation is most commonly Holder pasteurisation (milk heated for 30 minutes to 62.5°C), but other protocols such as high-temperature short-time (HTST) pasteurisation and newer technologies such as ultraviolet C (UVC) treatment show some promise. DHM processing renders the milk effectively sterile and in so doing destroys potentially harmful viruses, but is designed to be a balance between ensuring safety and maximising the range and function of the components after pasteurisation. The cellular and microbial content of milk is destroyed, and the bioactivity of some compounds, particularly enzymes such as lipase, is reduced. Therefore, DHM is not as nutritionally and developmentally complete as fresh or frozen maternal milk. However, DHM still contains a wide array of biologically active components that are not in infant formula. Such components include human milk oligosaccharides, which are unaffected by pasteurisation and growth factors such as epidermal growth factor, lactoferrin and lysozyme. Ongoing research is focusing on improving milk bank processes using simple, cost-effective interventions, such as nutritional supplementation for donors and improved transport and storage protocols.

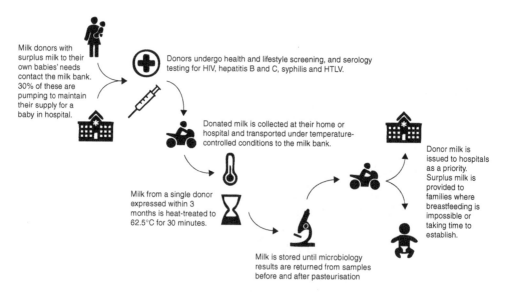

Figure 13.3 The pathway of milk through a human milk bank

How should donor milk be used?

According to the hierarchy of feeding choices recommended by the WHO, and supported by UNICEF and PATH, mother's own milk is always the first choice for feeding infants (PATH 2017). Several hospitals in the UK with in-house milk banks use DHM on a traffic light system, with priority given to the babies with the lowest birthweight and gestational ages, but equitable access for all babies in hospital when supplies of DHM are high. DHM will remain a rationed resource for several years to come in the UK, but with an increased evidence base and health economics rationale, as well as awareness raised by the Human Milk Foundation and UK Association for Milk Banking, wider access will come across the country as milk banks receive greater support. The context in which DHM should be considered is outlined in Figure 13.4, with the emphasis always on the support of mothers to establish their own supply.

Donor milk may lose some of the calorie content of MOM during processing. Growth is often perceived as a concern with the long-term use of DHM, and DHM may need supplementation with protein and multivitamins if used over a long duration. Currently, these are only available from a bovine milk-derived fortifier, and no independent studies have shown a clinical benefit to using newer human milk fortifiers. Full-term babies fed exclusively with human milk via clinical referral to the Hearts Milk Bank all grew according to expected rates, and developed normally (data pending publication, Bramer), but full-term babies do not have the high metabolic demands of preterm infants. It should be highlighted, though, that as a bridge to help a mother establish breastfeeding, the median duration of use for DHM on the NICU is 5 days. If DHM is fed as a supplement alongside MOM, the maternal microbiome is supported to be established by DHM components, such as oligosaccharides and lactoferrin (Cacho et al. 2017). The benefits of preserving an exclusive human milk diet to the baby in the longer term may exceed concerns about growth in the shorter term.

Room for improvement?

With increased resourcing into the milk bank infrastructure, evidence to target DHM use needs to be generated across multiple spheres, including the health economics of DHM use in different contexts, randomised controlled trials for DHM use in the context of supporting maternal breastfeeding, modelling potential use requirements to plan for scaling services and understanding the complexity of human milk composition changes and interindividual differences (John et al. 2019). It is likely that the true functional value of human milk will be completely separate from the number of calories and macronutrients provided, and entirely due to the individualised complexity of the thousands of bioactive factors – literally, the soup rather than the ingredients. Enhanced profiling of individual batches of donor milk is a research priority, and will form a large part of my working life for the next years to come.

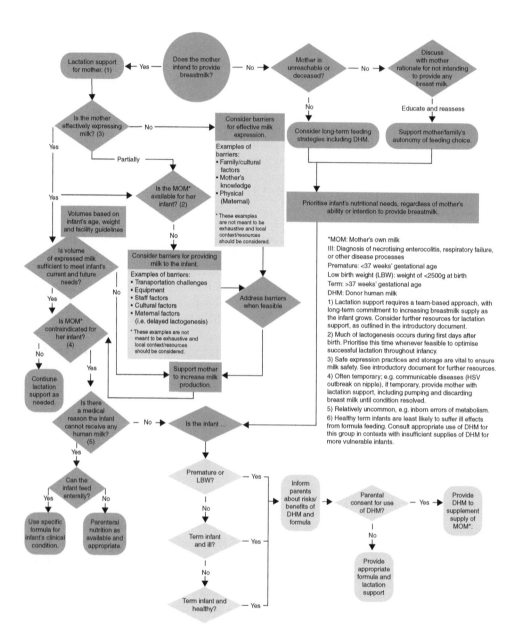

Figure 13.4 Decision-making tree for donor human milk

Source: Reproduced from PATH with permission: www.path.org/programs/maternal-newborn-child-health-and-nutrition/strengthening-human-milk-banking-resource-toolkit-4/.

References

Allin B, Long AM, Gupta A, Knight M, Lakhoo K; British Association of Paediatric Surgeons Congenital Anomalies Surveillance System Necrotising Enterocolitis Collaboration (2017) A UK wide cohort study describing management and outcomes for infants with surgical necrotising enterocolitis. *Sci Rep* 7:41149.

Allin BSR, Long AM, Gupta A, Lakhoo K, Knight M; British Association of Paediatric Surgeons Congenital Anomalies Surveillance System Necrotising Enterocolitis Collaboration (2018) One-year outcomes following surgery for necrotising enterocolitis: a UK-wide cohort study. *Arch Dis Child Fetal Neonatal Ed* 103(5):F461–6.

Arslanoglu S, Corpeleijn W, Moro G, Braegger C, Campoy C, Colomb V, Decsi T, Domellof M, Fewtrell M, Hojsak I, Mihatsch W, Mølgaard C, Shamir R, Turck D, van Goudoever J; ESPGHAN Committee on Nutrition (2013) Donor human milk for preterm infants: current evidence and research directions. *JPGN* 57:535–42.

BAPM (2016) The Use of Donor Human Expressed Breast Milk in Newborns: A Framework for Practice. www.bapm.org/resources/43-the-use-of-donor-human-expressed-breast-milk-in-newborn-infants-a-framework-for-practice-2016

Blesa M, Sullivan G, Anblagan D, Telford EJ, Quigley AJ, Sparrow SA et al. (2019) Early breast milk exposure modifies brain connectivity in preterm infants. *Neuroimage* 184:431–9.

Bode L (2012) Human milk oligosaccharides: every baby needs a sugar mama. *Glycobiology* 22(9):1147–62.

Boyd CA, Quigley MA, Brocklehurst P (2007) Donor breast milk versus infant formula for preterm infants: systematic review and meta-analysis. *Arch Dis Child Fetal Neonatal Ed* 92(3):F169–75.

Cacho NT, Harrison NA, Parker LA, Padgett KA, Lemas DJ, Marcial GE et al. (2017) Personalization of the microbiota of donor human milk with mother's own milk. *Front Microbiol* 8:1470.

Chowning R, Radmacher P, Lewis S, Serke L, Pettit N, Adamkin DH (2016) A retrospective analysis of the effect of human milk on prevention of necrotizing enterocolitis and postnatal growth. *J Perinatol* 36(3):221–4.

Coscia A, Peila C, Bertino E, Coppa GV, Moro GE, Gabrielli O et al. (2015) Effect of Holder pasteurisation on human milk glycosaminoglycans. *J Pediatr Gastroenterol Nutr* 60(1):127–30.

DeMarchis A, Israel-Ballard K, Mansen KA, Engmann C (2016) Establishing an integrated human milk banking approach to strengthen newborn care. *J Perinatol* 37(5):469–474.

de Rooy L, Hawdon J (2002) Nutritional factors that affect the postnatal metabolic adaptation of full-term small- and large-for-gestational-age infants. *Pediatrics* 109(3):E42.

Forbes JD, Azad MB, Vehling L, Tun HM, Konya TB, Guttman DS et al. (2018) Association of exposure to formula in the hospital and subsequent infant feeding practices with gut microbiota and risk of overweight in the first year of life. *JAMA Pediatr* 172(7):e181161.

Groer M, Duffy A, Morse S, Kane B, Zaritt J, Roberts S et al. (2014) Cytokines, chemokines, and growth factors in banked human donor milk for preterm infants. *J Hum Lact* 30(3):317–23.

Groer MW, Gregory KE, Louis-Jacques A, Thibeau S, Walker WA (2015) The very low birth weight infant microbiome and childhood health. *Birth Defects Res C Embryo Today* 105(4):252–64.

John A, Sun R, Maillart L, Schaefer A, Hamilton Spence E, Perrin MT (2019) Macronutrient variability in human milk from donors to a milk bank: implications for feeding preterm infants. *PLoS One* 14(1):e0210610.

Kair LR, Flaherman VJ (2017) Donor milk or formula: a qualitative study of postpartum mothers of healthy newborns. *J Hum Lact* 33(4):710–16.

Kair LR, Flaherman VJ, Newby KA, Colaizy TT (2015) The experience of breastfeeding the late preterm infant: a qualitative study. *Breastfeed Med* 10(2):102–6.

Kantorowska A, Wei JC, Cohen RS, Lawrence RA, Gould JB, Lee HC (2016) Impact of donor milk availability on breast milk use and necrotizing enterocolitis rates. *Pediatrics* 137(3):e20153123.

Kennedy J, Matthews A, Abbott L, Dent J, Weaver G, Shenker N (2017) Lactation following bereavement: how can midwives support women to make informed choices? *Midwifery Digest* 27(4):497–501.

Lewandowski AJ, Lamata P, Francis JM, Piechnik SK, Ferreira VM, Boardman H et al. (2016) Breast milk consumption in preterm neonates and cardiac shape in adulthood. *Pediatrics* 138(1).

Lin AE, Autran CA, Szyszka A, Escajadillo T, Huang M, Godula K et al. (2017) Human milk oligosaccharides inhibit growth of group B. *J Biol Chem* 292(27):11243–9.

Moossavi S, Azad MB (2019) Quantifying and interpreting the association between early-life gut microbiota composition and childhood obesity. *MBio* 10(1):2787–18.

NICE (2010). Donor Milk Banks: The Operation of Donor Milk Bank Services (CG 93). NICE. www.nice.org.uk/guidance/cg93

Niño DF, Sodhi CP, Hackam DJ (2016) Necrotizing enterocolitis: new insights into pathogenesis and mechanisms. *Nat Rev Gastroenterol Hepatol* 13(10):590–600.

O'Connor DL, Gibbins S, Kiss A, Bando N, Brennan-Donnan J, Ng E et al. (2016) Effect of supplemental donor human milk compared with preterm formula on neurodevelopment of very low-birth-weight infants at 18 months: a randomized clinical trial. *JAMA* 16(18):1897–905.

Parker LA, Cacho N, Engelmann C, Benedict J, Wymer S, Michael W et al. (2019) Consumption of mother's own milk by infants born extremely preterm following implementation of a donor human milk program: a retrospective cohort study. *J Pediatr* 211:33–8.

PATH (2017) Ensuring equitable access to human milk for all infants. A comprehensive approach to essential newborn care. Seattle: PATH.

Peila C, Moro GE, Bertino E, Cavallarin L, Giribaldi M, Giuliani F et al. (2016) The effect of Holder pasteurization on nutrients and biologically-active components in donor human milk: a review. *Nutrients* 8(8).

Quigley M, McGuire W (2014) Formula versus donor breast milk for feeding preterm or low birth weight infants. *Cochrane Database Syst Rev*. 4:CD002971.

Quigley M, Embleton ND, McGuire W (2018) Formula versus donor breast milk for feeding preterm or low birth weight infants. *Cochrane Database Syst Rev* 6:CD002971.

Renfrew MJ, Craig D, Dyson L, McCormick F, Rice S, King SE et al. (2009) Breastfeeding promotion for infants in neonatal units: a systematic review and economic analysis. *Health Technol Assess* 13(40):1–146, iii–iv.

Segal F (2019) *Mother Ship*. Chatto & Windus.

Triantis V, Bode L, van Neerven RJJ (2018) Immunological effects of human milk oligosaccharides. *Front Pediatr* 6:190.

Villamor-Martínez E, Pierro M, Cavallaro G, Mosca F, Kramer BW, Villamor E (2018) Donor human milk protects against bronchopulmonary dysplasia: a systematic review and meta-analysis. *Nutrients* 10(2).

Wilson E, Edstedt Bonamy AK, Bonet M, Toome L, Rodrigues C, Howell EA et al. (2018) Room for improvement in breast milk feeding after very preterm birth in Europe: results from the EPICE cohort. *Matern Child Nutr* 14(1).

Zhou J, Shukla VV, John D, Chen C (2015) Human milk feeding as a protective factor for retinopathy of prematurity: a meta-analysis. *Pediatrics* 136(6):e1576–86.

14 Breastfeeding a baby with health complications

Sandeep Kaur Jawanda, Helen Calvert and Pippa Hodge

> This chapter presents stories and guidance from a practitioner and mothers for supporting babies to breastfeed with cleft lip and palate, Down syndrome and congenital heart disease.
>
> It may be assumed that breastfeeding a baby with complications would present insurmountable difficulties. The stories shared by these mothers show difficulties may be overcome even though there are hurdles.
>
> The strength of women to fight for the best for their babies should not be ignored and they deserve to be supported.

Breastfeeding a baby with a cleft lip and palate

Sandeep Kaur Jawanda, GP partner and mother to a baby with a cleft palate

I was waiting for child number three to arrive, with the usual pregnancy-related worries that I'm sure most mums reproducing in the 21st century go through (Figure 14.1). Is everything going to be OK?

My daughter arrived but didn't cry. I knew immediately there was a problem. She looked strange, something was really odd, the crazy flow of hormones and adrenaline makes even a medic mum question herself. Then I put her to the breast, she looked to latch but couldn't. 'Its OK, each child is different, don't panic, stay calm, cortisol inhibits lactation, stay relaxed.' This was my inner monologue, fuelled more so by the junior midwife who thought I was clearly overreacting and casually came in and out of the room to ensure baby was OK. On the outside I gave a cool calm, experienced mum vibe, inside – I wanted to scream for someone to help, help me now, my baby isn't feeding, something is seriously wrong, my baby is starving!

I had expressed colostrum, the most raw and vulnerable time of a woman's life. Postpartum has no glamour, milking myself like a cow into a syringe to make sure baby doesn't starve, survival mode takes over. My sister held the syringe whilst I managed 0.2 mL, deflated, depressed, terrified.

Hours passed, still no latch, she couldn't physically do it, what was wrong? Her chin was non-existent, what looked like a tie, but not a tongue tie, gums. Be a mum not a doctor, I kept telling myself. Until they came to discharge us, when another more experienced midwife arrived for the newborn infant physical examination (NIPE). 'Be a mum, not a doctor, be a mum, not a doctor, she's not feeding, she's going to die, you're going to be held responsible, be a ... sod it!' 'Have you checked for a cleft palate?' I asked calmly, expecting a no. And there it happened, crash buzzer, in flood the doctors and crash team take over, suctioning, saturation monitors and the rest, a junior doctor explained it was massive, I swore, then came a general blur before being escorted to the neonatal ITU.

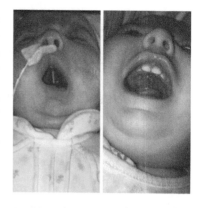

The diagnosis came over the next 24 hours: cleft palate with Pierre Robin syndrome, or sequence as it is often referred to now and a term I wish they had used at the time. Syndrome sounds terrifying with a definite connotation of long-term sequelae, even decreased life expectancy. I mentally prepared myself for the worst and when the cleft nurse confirmed it, I cried inconsolably.

Figure 14.1 Sandeep's daughter, born with a cleft palate, (left) before and (right) after the operation

She talked about feeding and I recall they told me I would never breastfeed my daughter. Devastated would be a massive understatement. I had breastfed my first-born, a journey itself, as he was born 4 lb at 33 weeks. I fed him for 2.5 years, only stopping because I fell pregnant. My second I breastfed for 8 months. To *not* breast-feed, simply put, wasn't an option I had considered, so now a stranger was telling me it wasn't possible.

Those few nights I had some form of grief reaction, it wasn't the diagnosis, I was pragmatic enough to realise. Actually I have a beautiful daughter, she is alive, get a grip, gain perspective and move on. It was the being unable to breastfeed, it broke me, I couldn't not breastfeed my child, such a strong urge I had to provide her with breastmilk. Let's make it clear, formula kept my boy and her alive on the neonatal units and it definitely has its place; I can only describe the overwhelming feeling. A black, depressed, dark time, sat contemplating my options. I couldn't do it, I couldn't *not* breastfeed, as much for my sanity as well as for her health – all of this whilst I sat in ITU with a poster stating the benefits of breastmilk versus formula. I felt terrible, so I decided to exclusively express. I turned to mums in the USA, who generally have shorter maternity leaves and do this much more often than I had heard of in the UK.

So I sized up my pump and went on my merry way. This was far from easy and it took the support of hundreds of strangers on closed social media group's, my husband, my family and friends to get me through. I expressed and fed my daughter with a nasogastric tube to 8 months, after which she had her cleft palate repair.

I expressed for a total of 12 months.

A few bumps along the way, a touch of mastitis, sepsis and infections, cancelled operations, but we made it. Gruelling, yes, rewarding, definitely, would I do it again – probably but with hesitation.

Breastfeeding and trisomy 21 (Down syndrome)

Pippa Hodge, co-ordinator, T21 Brighton and Hove

My third child, Leo (Figure 14.2), was born with antenatally diagnosed car-diac defects of Fallot's tetralogy/double-outlet right ventricle (DORV) and severe pulmonary stenosis, plus a surprise atrioventricular septal defect (AVSD) at 38+3. As per my 'hunch' plus a couple of clues along the way (I refused invasive testing), he also had 47 chromosomes – trisomy 21/Down syndrome. After initial Blalock–Thomas–Taussig (BTT) shunt surgery on his first full day of life, we entered a 'storm', with a pneumothorax, and then a pericardial effusion; he was a critically ill baby. Having breastfed my older two, I was determined that Leo would also receive breastmilk. I hand-expressed the colostrum,

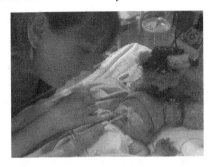

Figure 14.2 Leo

then switched to a manual pump, squeaking away in the paediatric intensive care unit (PICU), as close as possible to him without disturbing the wires and lines. It was hard. PICU is an incredibly tense environment; it's gut wrenching to leave your baby for the shortest while to eat or pee, let alone shower or sleep. Things change in an instant. Worry and fear definitely affected my let-down and flow. Where I had no option but to surrender my precious baby to the expertise of the surgical and PICU team and rely on them to keep him alive, seeing my colostrum and my milk going down the nasogastric tube gave me immense comfort. Promotion upstairs to the high-dependency unit came after 7 days, and we progressed slowly along the bays. Staff helped me by waking me so that I could express in the night and keep up the production.

Day 13: a landmark day – Leo's first day of breastfeeding! He was slow and tired, so after a few short stop/start feeds, we topped up expressed breastmilk (EBM) via his nasogastric tube. Day 14 dawned: good news! We were heading back to our local hospital for transitionary care. But as I undressed a sleepy Leo for his discharge weight, his arm was completely dark. It was a second, very serious pericardial effusion, but thanks to the fast-acting PICU team who drew 120 mL of fluid from the pericardial cavity around his tiny heart, Leo's life was saved again. It was then discovered that his thoracic duct had been compromised and he was switched to a medium-chain triglyceride (MCT) milk for 6 weeks.

Fast forward, and Leo, now just over 10 weeks old, was recovering in our local children's hospital from his third bronchiolitis episode. Meanwhile, our freezer was groaning with little bottles of EBM! It was a gruelling double regime – bottlefeeding the MCT whilst also trying to keep my milk flowing and stockpiling. The staff at the local hospital were pretty dismissive, and said it was extremely unlikely that a baby with Down syndrome who had been so unwell and had heart problems, and who would have poor muscle coordination and strength, would be able to feed, especially having had only one patchy day at the breast plus having been bottlefed for 6 weeks. 'Well, we won't know unless we try, will we?' I replied. I carefully lifted him from his cot, and after a couple of attempts he started to feed, and the tears rolled down my cheeks, as they are now, writing this. We continued with breastfeeding for a further 6 months, until his heart deterioration majorly impacted his stamina, and we switched to nasogastric feeding a high-calorie formula, in preparation for his open-heart surgery.

To you professionals, I ask you to stay open-minded. If mum planned to breastfeed, and trisomy 21 is diagnosed postnatally, encourage her to stick with her plan. Make sure she has support and guidance to achieve a good latch; encourage partners to keep her eating and drinking well; it may take time and there may need to be some topping up, but breastfeeding is important as it can help mum and baby (and partner) to find that extra closeness when coming to terms with unexpected news. Sometimes babies with trisomy 21 may have lower immunity or may have gone through an early surgery, so they especially need that wonderful elixir of antibodies. Lastly, the oral motor and coordination skills learned while breastfeeding form the building blocks for later speech and language development. So please, offer every encouragement and don't write breastfeeding (or EBM feeding) off for mums with babies who happen to be powered by an extra chromosome.

Breastfeeding with a congenital heart defect

Helen Calvert, parent and founder of Hospital Breastfeeding (www.facebook.com/hospitalbreastfeeding/)

My younger son, David (Figure 14.3), was born with hypoplastic left heart syndrome. This meant that he was transferred to Alder Hey Children's Hospital at a day old, and despite having had a caesarean section I requested I be discharged the same day so that I could be with him. Alder Hey was, therefore, also my maternity hospital. David was there until he was just over 3 weeks old. He had my milk from the day of his birth (via nasogastric tube) and I continued to express for him until he latched on at 4 weeks old and he breastfed until he was 4½ years old.

At 5 months old David had to have a second open heart surgery, and he was in hospital for just under a week. I was concerned about how I was going to be able to breastfeed him post-op, as he would be fully tubed up, including a couple of chest drains. In the event, I drop-fed him over the cot – leaving him lying down whilst I leant over him and popped my nipple into his mouth. Once his drains came out, I was then comfortable snuggling him again and normal feeding resumed.

I had promised myself that I would breastfeed him at least until his third open heart surgery was completed, but children being what they are, he self-weaned about 2 months before the procedure, at the age of 4½. I offered him a 'feed' when he was miserable in hospital that time around – he could have sucked for comfort, and I did still have some milk at that time. But he was adamant that he was done. David has always known his own mind!

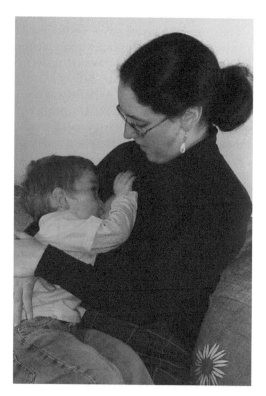

Figure 14.3 David

So, by our third major admission I wasn't a breastfeeding mother any more, but on the first two occasions that David was an inpatient at Alder Hey it was apparent to me that there was huge variation in breastfeeding knowledge amongst the nurses, and a huge variation in their interest in the subject. The speech and language therapist that we saw was a lovely lady but was clearly not trained in breastfeeding support, and neither was the dietitian, who confidently told me that we would be able to move David on to a 4-hour routine soon enough. As I said then, 'A 4-hour routine? For a breastfed baby?!' Or any baby for that matter. The overall impression I got was that breastfeeding was a lifestyle choice, which some nurses supported and others did not, but it was certainly not seen as an important part of paediatric care.

Following David's second admission, I contacted the hospital to see if they would be willing to discuss breastfeeding support. To their credit, Alder Hey has always been very open in talking to me about this subject. I was asked to contribute to the updating of their breastfeeding policy, and it was this experience that led me to start my #hospitalbreastfeeding campaign. I reached out on Twitter to the infant feeding and paediatric communities and I realised that I was not alone in my experiences. Paediatric wards and hospitals across the country have been pretty much left out of discussions of breastfeeding support.

There is lots of understanding and support for breastfeeding premature babies and those in the neonatal intensive care unit (NICU) which is wonderful, but many more babies who are born at term, or who get sick in their early years, are hospitalised whilst they are breastfed. Breastfeeding is *so* important for these babies. It's more than just nutrition – it's full of antibodies and is easy to digest – vital when a baby or child is sick. It can also provide great comfort for babies who are feeling unwell and in unfamiliar surroundings, undergoing different tests and procedures.

For David personally, breastfeeding was a fantastic way for him to regulate his temperature, something he struggled with as a cardiac baby. The other reason of course is that he was a normal baby who had been through a traumatic experience, and he wanted his mummy and the comfort of breastfeeding all the time. It is not all about food. David grew steadily and despite having a major heart defect we never had concerns about his food intake or growth.

Alder Hey is a regional centre for cardiac care and that really showed. Despite having top-class specialists for all other areas of medical care, when it comes to infant feeding the hospital leaves it very much down to the nurses and parents to muddle through together. And in saying this I am not singling out this wonderful hospital for criticism, because I know that most paediatric hospitals are the same.

The individual doctors and nurses were, in the main, fully supportive of breastfeeding, in the sense that they had no problem with me wanting to do it. My drop feeding David over the cot caused some consternation amongst the nurses, because apparently my body being used to feed my child is an uncomfortable thing for other adults and children to see on a paediatric ward, despite them having to view children in great pain, dragging chest drains around in baskets, screaming in terror at having to have bloods taken or walking around with fresh stitches on their chest. You would think the sight of a child being calmed and nurtured would be something to celebrate.

Of course, I know now just how little training about breastfeeding paediatricians, paediatric nurses and paediatric dietitians get. I have given talks to third-year nursing students who have been amazed by the information about breastfeeding being pain relief, infection control and its ability to raise a child's oxygen saturations. They are not taught these things as routine. However, parents assume health professionals are the experts, and will take their advice and not question it. I want to add in here that of course there are some people who are very knowledgeable about infant feeding, and some hospitals that provide excellent training to their staff. It's just unfortunately not standardised.

These issues are cultural, systemic and will take some time to address. But there are things that paediatricians and paediatric staff can do and consider immediately to better support breastfeeding as a part of children's medical care. Feeding at the breast will comfort a 4-year-old. Breastmilk will help to guard a 2-year-old against infection. A child of 3 can ingest breastmilk at the same time prior to surgery as could a baby. The functions of breastfeeding are not age-specific.

So, when it comes to supporting breastfeeding families, it would be so wonderful if all paediatric staff were aware of these functions. Not least because families are often not aware of these things themselves. So, a mother wanting to breastfeed her sick baby usually knows that it is the best form of nutrition for a child, but when faced with various medical realities she will start to lose faith in her body's ability to care for her baby. And if at that point staff are non-committal or even doubtful about breastfeeding, she will start to feel as though perhaps there is a medical alternative that is 'better' for her child. How wonderful would it be if all paediatric staff approached the mother (and the wider family who can support her to breastfeed) as part of the medical team? As a provider of medical care. And explained to her all the things that breastfeeding and breastmilk are giving to her child that can potentially improve that child's hospital experience and medical outcomes.

At this point I would like to talk about the 'pressure' to breastfeed. Because I know that many staff members are, quite rightly, worried about coming across as pressurising an already vulnerable mother to breastfeed her baby at a time when life is extremely stressful as that child is hospitalised. Supporting and respecting parental choice is vital, and breastfeeding can be very hard, especially in a hospital setting. I have not advocated and would never advocate insisting that mothers breastfeed or communicating with them in any way that makes them feel as though not doing so has somehow made them a failure as a parent. There will be families who are definite in their choice not to breastfeed and there will be families for whom breastfeeding is not an option. I have no interest in 'pressure' being placed on these families. However, we know that many babies and children are hospitalised when breastfeeding is already established. For these mothers, pressure is not the issue. The issue is empowerment.

In my experience with mothers, of all backgrounds and experiences, I can say this:

- Mothers feel guilty when they can't do something that everyone pretends is easy.
- Mothers feel pressurised when they are told they must do something that they think is hard, but everyone makes out is easy.
- Mothers feel empowered when they try to do something everyone says is hard, and they do it just a little bit.
- Mothers feel empowered when they are told that medical professionals need their help in caring for their child.

- Mothers feel reassured when the medical team emphasise that they support them and will provide them with the best knowledge and expertise to assist them.

It is how you ask, how you support, how you approach the issue that creates pressure or empowerment.

If I could only say one thing to paediatric doctors about infant feeding it is this: please do not assume that the nurses are providing the support. The nurses face the same barriers that you do: they often have very little infant feeding training, they have their own cultural and personal viewpoints on it, they have their own jobs to focus on and they are worried about 'getting it wrong'. If you would like your patients to benefit from the functions of breastfeeding, then please ensure that you are knowledgeable and that you know where to signpost families to for specialist support. Please do not rely on anyone else to do that.

We already know that doctors are amongst the groups of people who particularly struggle to breastfeed their own children, for all sorts of reasons. So, we also come upon the issue of cognitive dissonance when you are being asked to actively and confidently support something that you may not have been able to do, or chosen to do, yourself. I understand that this can create barriers. One of the most helpful things you can do for your patients and their families is to have a debrief yourself about your own infant feeding experiences.

I would like to close with a look at all the wonderful and positive things that I and other families have experienced in hospital settings when it comes to infant feeding.

Thank you to:

- any member of hospital staff who simply brings us a drink whilst we are feeding;
- any hospital that provides free meals to breastfeeding mothers. This can create controversy because it is seen a preferential treatment for those who can breast-feed, but of course it is simply providing free nutrition to the patient;
- the nursing staff who ask whether or not a mother wants privacy whilst she feeds her child, instead of assuming that she does or does not. For some mothers privacy is essential. For others, having the curtains pulled around them can feel shaming and isolating. Simply ask what a mother would prefer;
- all the health promotion teams who produce useful booklets or online information for families, often signposting to breastfeeding support outside of the hospital and helplines to call whilst a child is admitted. Knowing where to go for qualified support is incredibly helpful;
- all the doctors and nurses who take their own time to attend infant feeding conferences, read books like this one, attend training days or do online e-modules so that they can improve their infant feeding knowledge. We know how very busy you are, and we so appreciate you taking the time to find out how to best support your patient and their families;
- every healthcare professional who has not batted an eyelid when walking in on a breastfeeding mother or when a mother can only quiet and comfort her baby by feeding the child during a consultation;
- for not batting an eyelid when a mother has wanted to feed her child during a painful procedure;

- for not being grumpy when a mother yet again asks for a bottle of her expressed milk because her baby is feeding on demand. All we want to do is feed our children, provide them with comfort and give them everything that breastmilk and breastfeeding can provide to them, especially when they are sick.

Thank you to every healthcare professional who has made that easy for us.

15 Breastfeeding sick babies

Vicky Thomas

- Breastfeeding is even more important for ill children and their families than for healthy counterparts.
- If a baby can be fed, use breastmilk wherever possible.
- If a baby can be fed orally, feed at the breast wherever possible.
- When a baby cannot breastfeed, the mother will need skilled support with maintaining her milk supply so she can continue to express milk and will be able to continue breastfeeding at a later date if she wishes.
- The need for supplementation in ill babies must not be allowed to undermine the importance of breastfeeding and breastmilk as a key source of immune components, trophic effects on the gut and other major organs and in nurturing the parent–infant relationship.
- Consider a range of options if supplementing breastfeeding: at-breast supplementers, feeding tubes, bottles, cups, syringes, solid foods, high-calorie supplements and parenteral nutrition may all have a role.
- Centre the family in everything you do.

Breastfeeding has been identified as a key intervention in protecting the health of children across the world (Victora et al. 2016), yet those children who are already ill and who will arguably benefit the most from breastfeeding may be least likely to receive breastmilk if we regard it as an additional challenge rather than a cornerstone of good care. Our role as healthcare professionals is to support breastmilk feeding and breastfeeding wherever possible. Sadly, there is a dearth of literature on how to support breastfeeding in sick hospitalised children, but this chapter aims to offer stepping stones to clinicians working with families experiencing these challenges by reviewing theoretical principles, published literature and current custom and practice.

General principles for supporting breastfeeding families when the baby is unwell

There are very few absolute contraindications to breastfeeding or breastmilk feeding by bottle, cup, syringe or feeding tube. In fact, the World Health Organization (WHO) lists only rare metabolic conditions including galactosaemia, maple syrup urine disease and phenylketonuria (PKU) as absolute contraindications in the infant, and notes that some breastfeeding may be possible in PKU with careful monitoring (WHO 2009).

Additionally, breastfeeding is contraindicated where a baby has, or is suspected of having, severe combined immunodeficiency (SCID) and the mother is seropositive for cytomegalovirus (CMV), as this risks the baby contracting systemic CMV which can have devastating effects. If the mother's CMV status is not known, she should be encouraged to express and store her milk until her results are available, as if she is CMV-seronegative she will be able to resume breastfeeding and breastmilk feeding (Slatter 2019, personal communication). Expert opinion should be sought for any babies with other T-cell deficiencies or who are HIV positive.

In all other situations we must ask, and keep asking whenever the clinical condition changes:

- *When can we feed this baby breastmilk?*
- *When can this baby go to the breast?*
- *How can we support this family best?*

We should respect the family's choices at all times, but these choices need to be supported by education and practical assistance. There is a tendency to assume that families who are already dealing with the challenge of a sick baby will find breastfeeding an additional burden. In fact, parents in this situation often report that breastfeeding helps them to feel more empowered and connected to their child. At a time when a child may be too ill for normal care, handling and feeding by parents, ongoing support with breastfeeding and breastmilk feeding reinforce the crucial role that only they can play in their child's care and can be a link between parents and child.

Some babies with health challenges will need additional calories from supplementary feeds. We must not undermine breastfeeding by suggesting that breastmilk is inadequate – it is important to recognise that it is because of the child's health that more calories are needed than children require without this condition, and that breastmilk and breastfeeding provide nutritional and other impacts other feeds cannot.

When babies are too ill to feed at the breast, the mother should be supported to express regularly to maintain her milk supply, prevent engorgement and mastitis and provide milk for her baby when enteral feeding is possible. For a newborn this will mean expressing at least 8–10 times in 24 hours, including at least once between midnight and 6 a.m. For an exhausted and frightened parent, skilled lactation support may well be needed, especially if the baby is very young or has other risk factors for severe illness and breastfeeding is not fully established already. Clinicians who do not have expertise in lactation can help by being thoughtful, kind and supportive to parents in this position and recognising the challenges the family face and the unique role breastmilk can play in the child's recovery.

Physiological, immunological and psychological importance of breastfeeding sick children

The components of breastmilk are even more important for sick hospitalised children than their healthy counterparts. In particular we should consider the immune components, and trophic factors for the gut, brain and other organs which will be of special significance for unwell children.

Breastmilk feeding and breastfeeding have a key role in parent–infant bonding and attachment as well as supporting parental self-efficacy. Shah et al. (2012) showed that breastmilk or breastmilk feeding provides the best procedural pain relief for infants. While there are no large-scale data replicating this effect in older babies and children, common sense and clinician experience suggest that breastfeeding and breastmilk feeding are useful analgesic and distraction tools in these patient groups for blood taking, immunisation and cannulation.

In critically ill preterm babies, including those on ventilatory support, parent–infant skin-to-skin contact has been demonstrated to be safe and have beneficial effects including physiological stability (Jefferies 2012). While there are currently few data on sick older babies and children receiving skin-to-skin care, it is sensible to expect the same positive impacts in this group.

What health conditions cause babies and children to need support with breastfeeding?

We can broadly consider three groups of children in hospital with conditions impacting on breastfeeding:

1. premature and sick term infants who will usually be cared for in the neonatal unit and face their own distinct and well-recognised challenges;
2. babies who are usually well and have a transient acute illness which will temporarily impact on breastfeeding for hours or days;
3. those with chronic conditions which will impact on breastfeeding for weeks, months or years.

The latter two groups are usually cared for in specialist children's wards or hospitals which do not have recognised standards for breastfeeding support, in contrast to neonatal settings which should adhere to UNICEF Baby Friendly hospital standards.

Of course, this is an arbitrary distinction as the acute presentation may in fact be the start of a longer-term problem. Prematurity, in particular, can contribute to both short- and long-term difficulties with breastfeeding. It is useful to consider the challenges families face in these situations, and the overlap between them.

Babies in the neonatal unit

Chapter 2 covers the components and use of expressed human milk, both maternal and from milk banks. Here we consider how to transition these infants from expressed milk to breastfeeding. This will require an individual approach and experienced support. Practices described as baby-led, responsive and cue-based feeding focus on observing babies to interpret and respect their 'stop signs' rather than targeting specific volumes of feed and are becoming more prevalent. These do not result in reduced weight gain or delays in attaining full oral feeding and may reduce long-term feeding problems (Shaker 2013; Carrierfenster et al. 2018). Skin-to-skin care will help the baby recognise and respond to the cues provided by the mother's body and support physiological stability. Traditionally it was thought that babies under the age of 34 weeks' gestation were unlikely to manage oral feeding but babies from 29 weeks' gestation have been tried at the breast in order to build the feeding skills needed (Nyqvist 2008).

Babies and older children in children's wards and hospitals

Acute conditions which may require support with breastfeeding

RESPIRATORY PROBLEMS, ESPECIALLY CROUP, BRONCHIOLITIS AND PNEUMONIA

Acute respiratory conditions are the most common reasons for the admission of infants to hospital, and admission rates for these conditions are rising (Keeble and Kossarova 2017). Some babies with these conditions, particularly bronchiolitis, will be admitted to the paediatric intensive care unit for respiratory support, including endotracheal intubation and mechanical ventilation. Breathless babies can struggle to feed due to the challenge of coordinating sucking and swallowing when tachypnoeic, and significantly reduced feeding is one of the criteria for admission in bronchiolitis. In a medical culture which sees formula feeding as the default, clinicians can find it difficult to assess whether a breastfed infant is taking adequate milk. Clinical assessment and the parents' opinion are key; if the parents feel the baby's feeding is significantly disrupted, this should be taken seriously. Evidence of dehydration should be rapidly assessed and treated appropriately (see below).

Bronchiolitis symptoms usually last approximately 7–10 days, peaking at 3–5 days. At the nadir, the baby may need to be fed with a nasogastric or orogastric feeding tube either as bolus or continuous feeds. If the baby is very unwell, enteral feeds may need to be stopped entirely and intravenous fluids given as a full stomach can contribute to respiratory distress. Usually the baby will need only 50–75% of the normal fluid intake. If the baby is distressed by stopping feeds, skin-to-skin contact or comfort feeding at the breast as tolerated may help to settle this. The use of a dummy can be considered but should be discussed with the family if this is not their normal routine. Babies can usually be trusted to recognise their own limits and will feed or carry out non-nutritive sucking at the breast as is safe for them. If the baby is well enough to be held, tube feeds can be carried out while a parent or staff member holds the infant.

Once the baby starts to recover there is no need to transition to bottles to check the infant can tolerate a set volume of milk before trying the baby at the breast and this may in fact be counterproductive. Simply allow the baby to feed as s/he chooses at the breast and monitor clinically. The approaches described in the section on babies in the neonatal unit (see above) can also be applied to these babies when resuming feeds. Bronchiolitis can disrupt breastfeeding relationships (Helibronner et al. 2017) and it is important to try to minimise iatrogenic aspects of this.

GASTROENTERITIS, INCLUDING SHOCK AND DEHYDRATION

Gastroenteritis is less common in breastfed infants and children and so clinicians are often less confident in managing these babies. It is firstly necessary to assess for shock or dehydration as per National Institute for Health and Care Excellence (NICE) guidance (NICE 2009) (Figure 15.1). Shock should be treated with intravenous fluid boluses as required to replace an appropriate circulating fluid volume, followed by careful rehydration to make up the deficit over 48 hours. Children who are dehydrated but not shocked should be rehydrated enterally as this is more physiological and reduces the risk of iatrogenic hyponatraemia. This may entail the use of oral rehydration salts (ORS) via mouth or enteral feeding tube. Breastfed infants can continue to breastfeed throughout rehydration. A child who is vomiting repeatedly but not

Assessing dehydration in children under 5 years

Use this table to detect clinical dehydration and shock during remote and face-to-face assessments
Adapted from 'Diarrhoea and vomiting in children' (NICE clinical guideline 84). The quick reference guide and full guidance are available from: www.nice.org.uk/CG84

	No clinically detectable dehydration	Clinical dehydration	Clinical shock
		Increasing severity of dehydration →	
Symptoms (remote and face-to-face assessments)	Appears well	Appears to be unwell or deteriorating	–
	Alert and responsive	Altered responsiveness (for example, irritable, lethargic)	Decreased level of consciousness
	Normal urine output	Decreased urine output	–
	Skin colour unchanged	Skin colour unchanged	Pale or mottled skin
	Warm extremities	Warm extremities	Cold extremities
Signs (face-to-face assessments)	Alert and responsive	Altered responsiveness (for example, irritable, lethargic)	Decreased level of consciousness
	Skin colour unchanged	Skin colour unchanged	Pale or mottled skin
	Warm extremities	Warm extremities	Cold extremities
	Eyes not sunken	Sunken eyes	–
	Moist mucous membranes (except after a drink)	Dry mucous membranes (except for 'mouth breather')	–
	Normal heart rate	Tachycardia	Tachycardia
	Normal breathing pattern	Tachypnoea	Tachypnoea
	Normal peripheral pulses	Normal peripheral pulses	Weak peripheral pulses
	Normal capillary refill time	Normal capillary refill time	Prolonged capillary refill time
	Normal skin turgor	Reduced skin turgor	–
	Normal blood pressure	Normal blood pressure	Hypotension (decompensated shock)

Box 1 At increased risk of dehydration:
- Children younger than 1 year, especially those younger than 6 months
- infants who were of low birth weight
- children who have passed six or more diarrhoeal stools in the past 24 hours
- children who have vomited three times or more in the past 24 hours
- children who have not been offered or have not been able to tolerate supplementary fluids before presentation
- infants who have stopped breastfeeding during the illness
- children with signs of malnutrition.

Suspect hypernatraemic dehydration if there are any of the following:
- jittery movements
- increased muscle tone
- hyperreflexia
- convulsions
- drowsiness or coma.

Laboratory investigations:
- Do not routinely perform blood biochemistry.
- Measure plasma sodium, potassium, urea, creatinine and glucose concentrations if:
  - intravenous fluid therapy is required **or**
  - there are symptoms or signs suggesting hypernatraemia.
- Measure venous blood acid–base status and chloride concentration if shock is suspected or confirmed.

Interpret symptoms and signs taking into account risk factors for dehydration (see box 1). More numerous and more pronounced symptoms and signs of clinical dehydration indicate greater severity. For clinical shock, one or more of the symptoms and/or signs listed would be present. Dashes (–) indicate that these clinical features do not specifically indicate shock. Symptoms and signs with red flags (🚩) may help to identify children at increased risk of progression to shock. If in doubt, manage as if there are symptoms and/or signs with red flags.

Figure 15.1 Assessing dehydration in children under 5 years
Source: NICE (2009)

dehydrated is often subjected to a 'fluid challenge' of small volumes of ORS via bottle, cup or syringe to ensure s/he can tolerate oral fluids and break the 'drink–vomit' cycle often seen when a thirsty child consumes fluid which makes a rapid reappearance. There is no need to stop breastfeeding and substitute with ORS or make a mother express breastmilk to attempt this in a breastfed child. If a fluid challenge is felt necessary in a breastfed child, some mothers find it helpful to breastfeed for a short period and then distract the baby briefly to allow the milk to be absorbed before allowing a return to the breast. The periods of breastfeeding can gradually increase in length as the baby tolerates milk and remains hydrated.

JAUNDICE AND OTHER LIVER PROBLEMS

Liver disease is not a contraindication to breastfeeding. Babies who are jaundiced should be assessed as per NICE (2016). In particular, experienced and skilled breastfeeding support should be sought to ensure the jaundice is not related to inadequate milk intake, and to support ongoing breastfeeding and/or expressing if the baby requires intensive phototherapy. Phototherapy should be delivered with the least possible interference in breastfeeding and skin-to-skin contact.

SEVERE INFECTION OF ANY ORIGIN, INCLUDING SEPSIS AND MENINGITIS

This is not a contraindication to breastfeeding or breastmilk feeding and, if the baby is alert enough to feed, responsive breastfeeding can continue throughout the illness, or be resumed once the baby recovers. In the interim, tube feeding or intravenous fluids may be required as above.

PAIN OR DYSFUNCTION OF THE MOUTH AND THROAT

In tonsillitis and other bacterial and viral infections of the mouth, including hand-foot-and-mouth disease and herpes simplex virus (HSV) gingivostomatitis, breastfeeding may provide physical and psychological comfort. If the child refuses to drink, topical and oral analgesia should be given. Yoghurts, ice cream and ice lollies can be used to provide hydration and soothe the mouths of older infants and toddlers. Expressed breastmilk can be frozen into ice lollies. Standard hand hygiene precautions will reduce the risk of transmission of the infection to the mother. If the child is unable to feed orally, tube feeding or intravenous maintenance fluids should be given.

ACUTE SURGICAL ISSUES AFFECTING THE GUT

Congenital malformations such as tracheo-oesophageal fistula, gastroschisis and exomphalos and acute illnesses including necrotising enterocolitis (NEC) can result in babies being unable to have oral or enteral feeds while they await or recover from surgery. Breastmilk remains the optimal feed for these babies and breastfeeding is the ideal way of delivering it when safe to feed by mouth.

ANAESTHESIA

The Academy of Breastfeeding Medicine (2012) recommends that breastfeeding and breastmilk feeding are withheld for 4 hours prior to anaesthesia, with clear fluids permitted up to 2 hours before. Local protocols may differ.

ACUTE ILLNESS OR INJURY AFFECTING THE LIMBS OR THE NERVOUS SYSTEM

Babies who are injured or have illnesses causing pain and/or limitation of movement of their limbs may need additional support with comfortable and effective positioning and attachment for breastfeeding. Regular analgesia and skilled experienced support are crucial.

Long-term conditions which may require support with breastfeeding

CONGENITAL HEART DISEASE (CHD)

Babies with heart abnormalities may face particular challenges with breastfeeding but breastmilk is a lifesaving intervention for this group of infants, who are especially at risk from NEC, poor growth, feed intolerance and swallow issues (Davis and Spatz 2019). Barriers include delays in initiating enteral, oral and at-breast feeds due to clinical instability and clinician anxiety, and lack of support for mothers in expressing and breastfeeding. Key interventions include:

1. education of families regarding the importance of breastmilk;
2. initiation of breastfeeding (or expressing if the infant is unable to breastfeed) within 1 hour of birth;
3. ongoing support for expressing;
4. early skin-to-skin contact;
5. oral care with colostrum if the baby is not able to breastfeed;
6. non-nutritive sucking at the breast;
7. recognition that breastfeeding results in more physiological stability than bottlefeeding for infants with CHD;
8. use of skimmed human milk if possible rather than specialist formula for infants who develop chylothorax as weight gain is better with skimmed human milk.

Immediate pre- and post-feed weights can be a useful way of assessing milk intake at the breast. See Chapter 14 for the experiences of a mum whose baby had a heart defect.

LONG-TERM RESPIRATORY CONDITIONS

Any respiratory condition can make oral feeding of any kind more challenging as it is harder to coordinate breathing and feeding. Children with breathing problems often have additional energy requirements and may require supplementation. Breastfeeding remains the optimal feeding method. Cystic fibrosis (CF) is an example of this: breastfeeding does not compromise growth and is associated with fewer infections and respiratory problems (Jadin et al. 2011). Pancreatic enzyme supplements may be recommended to improve feed tolerance and increase weight.

Airway anomalies may make swallowing unsafe and necessitate tube feeding. It is possible to breastfeed a child with a tracheostomy but it may require skilled multi-disciplinary support – Grainne Evans has written a moving and useful account of her daughter's experience (Evans 2018).

COMPLEX SURGICAL CONDITIONS AFFECTING THE GUT

For congenital abnormalities of the gut, or those acquired in early infancy, breastmilk remains the best-tolerated and optimal feed. Some babies with complex anomalies, in particular long-gap oesophageal atresia, will have a prolonged period of being unable to feed by mouth as their gastrointestinal tract is in discontinuity. 'Sham feeds' by breast or bottle can be given by mouth, drained from the upper oesophageal pouch to prevent aspiration into the lungs and then re-fed into the gastrostomy. This aims to help the infant learn to associate feeding by mouth with the sensation of stomach fullness and reduce oral aversion. It may be recommended for the mother to express before undertaking initial sham feeding at the breast so the baby does not need to contend with a full breast.

CHRONIC KIDNEY DISEASE

In most children with chronic kidney disease (CKD), breastmilk is the ideal enteral fluid due to its low renal solute load and low potassium, although sometimes a specialist formula even lower in potassium is required. If babies need additional calories due to their clinical condition, it is possible to use breastmilk fortifier or supplementary feeds. When detailed fluid balance documentation is essential, some sources suggest feeding expressed breastmilk via bottle or enteral tube (Samman and Secker 2014), although there are alternative ways of assessing the child, including clinical examination, frequent weighing and biochemical assessment. If the baby must be fluid-restricted, it is usually possible to breastfeed for at least 5–10 minutes and then give a known volume of expressed breastmilk or formula milk.

ABNORMAL TONE AND MOVEMENT

Babies who are especially floppy or stiff, or who have reduced movement in some or all limbs as a result of an underlying neurological condition, will benefit from additional support with breastfeeding positioning and sucking skills. Some parents are incorrectly told that conditions such as Down syndrome preclude breastfeeding, but skilled support can facilitate breastfeeding in these babies. If there is any concern over the safety of their swallow, specialist assessment should be sought.

CLEFT LIP AND/OR PALATE AND ANY OTHER STRUCTURAL ANOMALY OF THE FACE OR MOUTH

See Chapter 14 for the experience of a GP mum.

INSULIN-DEPENDENT DIABETES MELLITUS

It is possible to breastfeed a child with insulin-dependent diabetes mellitus. There is a useful protocol for this (Miller et al. 2017) which advises on average milk volumes consumed per day by age of infant and the carbohydrate count of breastmilk to aid with insulin dosing.

CONGENITAL ADRENAL HYPERPLASIA

Babies with this endocrine condition resulting in reduced production of endogenous steroid can breastfeed safely, though may require saline supplements in addition to compensate if salt wasting is present.

ONCOLOGICAL DIAGNOSES AND TREATMENTS

Children may gain comfort and immunological support by continuing breastfeeding throughout a diagnosis of, and treatment for, cancer. Anecdotally, breastfed oncology patients tolerate chemotherapy and radiotherapy well and seem to have fewer problems with mucositis.

References

Academy of Breastfeeding Medicine (2012) ABM clinical protocol #25: recommendations for preprocedural fasting for the breastfed infant: "NPO" guidelines. *Breastfeed Med* 7:197–202.

Carrierfenster K, Rue-Donlon C, Khalak R (2018) Getting to full feeds faster in the NICU using cue-based feeding. *Pediatrics* 141(1): meeting abstract.

Davis JA, Spatz DL (2019) Human milk and infants with congenital heart disease: a summary of current literature supporting the provision of human milk and breastfeeding. *Adv Neonat Care* 19(3):212–18.

Evans G (2018) Breastfeeding with a tracheostomy. Part two. *Against the Odds* [Blog]. https://birthingandbreastfeeding.wordpress.com/2013/08/10/breastfeeding-tracheostomies-tears-and-triummphs-part-two

Helibronner C, Roy E, Hadchouel A, Jebali S, Smii S, Masson A, Renolleau S, Rigourd V (2017) Breastfeeding disruption during hospitalisation for bronchiolitis in children: a telephone survey. *BMJ Paediatr Open* 1:e000158.

Jadin SA, Wu GS, Zhang Z, Shoff SM, Tippets BM, Farrell PM … Lai HJ (2011) Growth and pulmonary outcomes during the first 2 y of life of breastfed and formula-fed infants diagnosed with cystic fibrosis through the Wisconsin Routine Newborn Screening Program. *Am J Clin Nutr* 93(5):1038–47.

Jefferies AL (2012) Canadian Paediatric Society, Fetus and Newborn Committee. Kangaroo care for the preterm infant and family. *Paediatr Child Health* 17(3):141–3.

Keeble E, Kossarova L (2017) Emergency hospital care for children and young people. Nuffield Trust. www.nuffieldtrust.org.uk/files/2018-10/1540142848_qualitywatch-emergency-hospital-care-children-and-young-people-full.pdf

Miller D, Mamilly L, Fourtner S, Rosen-Carole C; Academy of Breastfeeding Medicine (2017) ABM clinical protocol# 27: breastfeeding an infant or young child with insulin-dependent diabetes. *Breastfeed Med* 12(2):72–6.

NICE (2009) Diarrhoea and vomiting caused by gastroenteritis in under 5s: diagnosis and management. www.nice.org.uk/guidance/cg84/chapter/1-Guidance#assessing-dehydration-and-shock-2

NICE (2016) Jaundice in newborn babies under 28 days. CG 98. www.nice.org.uk/guidance/CG98

Nyqvist KH (2008) Early attainment of breastfeeding competence in very preterm infants. *Acta Paediatr* 97:776–81.

Samaan S, Secker D (2014) Oral feeding challenges in infants with chronic kidney disease. *Infant Child Adolesc Nutr* 6:164–71.

Shah PS, Herbozo C, Aliwalas LL, Shah VS (2012) Breastfeeding or breast milk for procedural pain in neonates. *Cochrane Database Syst Review* 12:CD004950.

Shaker CS (2013) Cue-based feeding in the NICU; using the infant's communication as a guide. *Neonat Network* 32:404–8.

Victora CG, Bahl R, Barros AJD, França GVA, Horton S, Krasavec J ... Rollins NC (2016) Breastfeeding in the 21st century: epidemiology, mechanisms, and lifelong effect. *Lancet* 387:475–90.

WHO (2009) Acceptable medical reasons for use of breast-milk substitutes. https://apps.who.int/iris/bitstream/handle/10665/69938/WHO_FCH_CAH_09.01_eng.pdf?ua=1

16 Infant feeding in emergencies – what doctors need to know

Helen Gray

- Support breastfeeding mothers to keep breastfeeding.
- Support mothers who are mixed feeding to increase breastfeeding and reduce the need for formula and bottles.
- For formula-feeding families, ensure access to suitable formula supplies and adequate clean water, along with clean preparation and milk storage facilities.
- In a longer-term emergency situation, some mothers may choose to relactate and will require specialist support.

Disasters can happen in any country, and the UK is no exception – recent years have seen storms, flooding, widespread water contamination, and terrorist attacks. The health services are a key component of resilience planning and response. In any disaster, infants, toddlers and their mothers are among the most vulnerable. Formula-fed infants are at even higher risk, because they lack the immune protection provided by breastfeeding, and they are dependent on access to clean water, facilities and supplies for the safe preparation of formula and bottles (Gribble 2011). What do doctors and other healthcare professionals need to know about infant feeding in emergency situations?

International operational guidance on infant and young child feeding in emergencies is available and should form the basis of resilience planning (Infant Feeding in Emergencies Core Group 2017). Currently there is no national guidance in the UK on infant and young child feeding in emergencies. The UK received a score of 0/10 on emergency planning in the World Breastfeeding Trends Initiative assessment (Gray et al. 2016). Emergency and disaster planning has been devolved to local resilience forums. Many area resilience plans do not include infants and young children or breastfeeding women, as they do not fall under the definition of 'vulnerable' groups in the Civil Contingencies guidance (Cabinet Office Civil Contingencies Secretariat 2008).

Risks to infants and young children in an emergency in the UK include:

- lack of breastfeeding, early weaning and mixed feeding contributing to increased risks of illness and infection (Victora et al. 2016);
- pathogens in the water and bacteria in powdered formula can cause illness if water is not boiled and used at 70°C (Gribble 2011);
- lack of suitable facilities and electricity to boil water, clean bottles, prepare and store formula safely: contamination of bottles, teats and preparation surfaces increases risks of infection and illness. Breast pumps can also be very difficult to clean and sterilise in disaster conditions;

- lack of clean water: families require an estimated 24 litres of clean water every day to safely clean bottles and prepare powdered formula, and 12 litres every day if using ready-to-feed formula (Gribble and Berry 2011). In the UK, the water regulator requires water companies to distribute only 10 litres of water per person per day in the event of an interruption in water supply (www.ofwat.gov. uk/households/supply-and-standards/supply-interruptions/);
- lack of trained support for breastfeeding mothers;
- indiscriminate donations of inappropriate or free formula (Gribble 2016);
- the use of processed convenience foods for toddlers such as baby food pouches or toddler formulas can leave families reliant on expensive processed foods, often high in sugar, for their young children after the emergency is over (DeYoung et al. 2018);
- poor organisation of family spaces, lack of privacy, queues for food and services can separate families and reduce opportunities for mothers to feed their babies;
- families where breastfeeding is the most fragile may also be those who are most reliant on rest centres. These families may find that breastfeeding is more easily disrupted during the emergency, magnifying health inequalities.

Preparation and planning

Each local area should have a basic needs assessment, including the number of local infants and children, their ages and whether they are breastfed, to assist in planning for emergencies. Local authorities, public health (for example, Public Health England (PHE) fingertips child health data; https://fingertips.phe.org.uk/profile/child-health-profiles) and maternity units will all have some of this information if there is no comprehensive local needs assessment. Collaboration is essential to meet families' medical and feeding needs (American Academy of Pediatrics 2015).

Key points for supporting breastfeeding families in an emergency

- Keep families together and create safe parenting spaces with counselling, food and water available.
- It is important to rapidly assess how many infants and young children are currently being breastfed and how many require support with safe formula feeding. This will quickly establish what resources, skilled help and facilities are needed.
- Breastfeeding mothers may need skilled lactation support to overcome any challenges and continue breastfeeding. Mothers who are mixed feeding can be supported to increase breastfeeding and reduce their reliance on formula. In long-term emergency situations, some mothers may choose to relactate with skilled support. Assure mothers that human milk provides significant nutrition for the first year of life and beyond, even when complementary foods are not available.
- Formula-feeding families will need a safe source of formula and somewhere clean to prepare it. A 'milk kitchen' facility with separate distribution, hygienic preparation and storage facilities is essential. Only use powdered formula if clean or boiled water is available at 70°C, otherwise use ready–to-feed liquid first-stage formula.
- Appropriate supplies should be planned for local rest centres, such as stage 1 infant formula (suitable for most infants up to 1 year), cups, bottles and teats,

along with suitable equipment for preparation, sterilisation and storage. Small cups are safest and easiest to clean.

- Assess and support the hydration and nutrition of both mother and infant. It is important that separate queues and arrangements for food distribution are in place for families with infants and young children. Infants and young children have specific nutritional needs, as do pregnant and lactating mothers.
- Monitor maternal health: breastfeeding women should be appropriately immunised. If medication is required refer to national and international guidelines for specific diseases (e.g. the UK Drugs in Lactation Advisory Service (UKDILAS) and the Breastfeeding Network's Drugs in Breastmilk Service)
- Advocate for breastfeeding and for safe infant feeding practices among relief agencies and workers, who may not be aware of its importance.
- While the public is often keen to donate milk for babies, this can cause significant problems for rescue workers who have to sort, store and distribute it. Focus on supporting mothers to increase their milk supply where possible, and donate funds rather than formula.

Source: American Academy of Pediatrics (2015) and
Infant Feeding in Emergencies Core Group (2017)

References

American Academy of Pediatrics (2015) Infant Feeding in Disasters and Emergencies: Breastfeeding and Other Options. www.aap.org/en-us/advocacy-and-policy/aap-health-initiatives/breast feeding/documents/infantnutritiondisaster.pdf

Cabinet Office Civil Contingencies Secretariat (2008) Identifying People Who Are Vulnerable in a Crisis: Guidance for Emergency Planners and Responders. www.gov.uk/government/publications/identifying-people-who-are-vulnerable-in-a-crisis-guidance-for-emergency-planners-and-responders

DeYoung S, Chase J, Branco M, Park B (2018) The effect of mass evacuation on infant feeding: the case of the 2016 Fort McMurray wildfire. *Matern Child Health J* 30(3).

Gray H, Meynell C, Spiro A, Wise P et al. (2016) *World Breastfeeding Trends Initiative UK Report.* https://ukbreastfeedingtrends.files.wordpress.com/2017/03/wbti-uk-report-2016-part-1-14-2-17.pdf

Gribble K (2011) Mechanisms behind breastmilk's protection against, and artificial baby milk's facilitation of, diarrhoeal illness. *Breastfeed Rev* 19(2):19–26.

Gribble K (2016) Why breastfeeding mothers request and use infant formula. https://anthrol actology.com/2016/01/16/why-breastfeeding-mothers-request-and-use-donated-infant-formula/

Gribble K, Berry N (2011) Emergency preparedness for those who care for infants in developed country contexts. *Int Breastfeed J* 6:16.

Infant Feeding in Emergencies Core Group (2017) Infant and young child feeding in emergencies: Operational guidance for emergency relief staff and programme managers, version 3. www. ennonline.net/operationalguidance-v3-2017

Victora CG, Bahl R, Barros AJ (2016) Breastfeeding in the 21st century: epidemiology, mechanisms, and lifelong effect. *Lancet* 387(10017):475–90.

17 What GPs need to know about breastmilk substitutes

Helen Crawley

- Most healthy infants in the UK who are not fully breastfed need a first infant formula throughout the first year of life as their breastmilk substitute (BMS).
- All infant formula must have a similar nutritional composition by law. Manufacturers often add unnecessary ingredients to make claims for the superiority of their product. This can lead to financial hardship amongst families who believe that by paying more money they are doing the best for their baby.
- Many products on the market are not needed: for example, hungry baby formula, follow-on formula, goodnight milk, comfort milks and milks marketed for children over 1 year of age.
- It is useful to know where to access information on infant milks if families want to know whether products are halal-certified or vegetarian, how the costs compare and what evidence there is to support any claims made. This can all be accessed at www.firststepsnutrition.org/composition-claims-and-costs.
- Some specialist formulas are available without prescription and there is concern that these encourage families to self-medicate their infants and promote the view that many normal infant feeding behaviours require specialist treatment. Anti-reflux milks and lactose-free formula should only be used under medical supervision.
- The advertising and marketing of BMS allow information to be given to health professionals that is 'scientific and factual' but there is no independent verification if this is the case, and adverts for many products, including specialist formula, have been reported to be misleading.
- Powdered infant milks are not sterile and making up infant formula safely to protect infants from bacterial infection remains essential.

Introduction

The majority of infants in the UK will be given a BMS in the first year of life, and some will continue to be given these in the second year and beyond. The names we use for these BMS vary, but many people use the term infant formula to cover a whole range of products that are regulated in different ways in the UK. One of the constant complaints heard by health professionals is that 'no one told me what sort of formula to buy' and there are myths that staff trained in Unicef UK Baby Friendly-accredited settings are 'not allowed' to support formula-feeding families. Much of the confusion comes from the placing on the market of a lot of unnecessary products, and the fact that global marketing restrictions which aim to protect families from misleading claims about products are not enforced in the UK. As part of the Unicef UK Baby Friendly Initiative staff must demonstrate support to formula-feeding families and can of course talk about different types of formula, but should not highlight particular brands. The same is true for all health professionals who can talk about types of formula but should not promote brands. Sadly the heavy promotion of some brand names means that they become synonymous with the type of product, much as the words Hoover and Sellotape are commonly used to denote product type. It is important that health professionals don't fall into this marketing trap. The simple message that all health professionals need is that the majority of infants only require a first infant formula (often called stage 1) for the whole of the first year, and that all infant formula on the market must be a similar nutritional composition by law.

Whilst the information that both families and health professionals need is not complicated, the BMS company-funded training and advertising aimed at GPs and other health professionals encourage the promotion of more expensive brands and types of milks, so it is no surprise that the basic messages get lost in all the noise. It goes without saying that the marketing and advertising of BMS undermine breastfeeding in the UK, which is the 11th biggest formula market in the world, highlighting how low our breastfeeding rates are. Manufacturers spend over £20 per baby born in the UK each year advertising formula brands. The International Code of Marketing of Breastmilk Substitutes (WHO 1981) (and subsequent World Health Assembly resolutions) aims to protect families and health workers from conflict of interest, and the Code is clear that companies selling foods for infants and young children should not make donations to health workers or professional associations or sponsor meetings of health professionals or scientific meetings. Whilst we have some, but not all, of the Code in UK law, all those working in Unicef UK Baby Friendly-accredited neonatal, maternity, community and university settings abide by the Code, and the number of accredited settings is rapidly increasing, supported by the NHS plan and many regional initiatives.

'Closer to breastmilk?'

For avoidance of doubt, you cannot create a BMS that is 'close to breastmilk' – it is impossible to recreate breastmilk. Breastmilk is nutritionally suited to the human infant and contains hundreds of unique components and living cells to protect infants from infection and to aid development. 'Structurally identical' components to factors found in breastmilk can be made in laboratories but are unlikely to have the same functional capacity and most of the components much lauded in advertising of products have been shown to be unnecessary additions to infant formula (and a potential burden on a young child's metabolism). All infant formulas have to be of a similar nutritional composition to comply with EU regulations. If a substance was found that was agreed to be beneficial for infant health that could be added to infant formula, it would be in all infant formula by law.

So what do you need to know about breastmilk substitutes?

What counts as a breastmilk substitute?

The World Health Organization (WHO 2017) defines BMS as any milks (or products that could be used to replace milks) that are specifically marketed for feeding infants and young children up to the age of 3 years, including infant formula, follow-on formula, specialist milks and toddler milks. BMS also include any foods marketed to infants during the first 6 months of life, feeding bottles and teats.

What products are available on the UK market?

Infant formula can be made from cows' milk or goats' milk protein, soya protein or hydrolysed proteins. Some may be made from organic ingredients but the majority of products used are from two companies and are based on cows' milk protein (Cow & Gate and Aptamil (Danone Nutricia) and SMA (Nestlé)). In order to segment the market SMA and Aptamil offer premium versions of their branded infant formula, but there are no agreed benefits for using these and they can cost a family £30–40 a month more than a perfectly suitable cheaper infant formula. One brand of soya-based infant formula is available in the UK but it is recommended that this is used only under medical supervision because of concerns about the phyto-oestrogens present.

Follow-on formulas are covered by specific regulations but are agreed by all health bodies as unnecessary. Producing a very similar-looking follow-on formula product allows companies to advertise their brand. In the USA where there are no restrictions on advertising infant formula, there are no follow-on formulas. Families should be encouraged to use a first infant formula throughout the first year as this is the product that is agreed to be the best alternative to breastmilk nutritionally.

Foods for special medical purposes are also regulated under separate legislation, and this specifies that all products in this category should used under medical supervision. Despite this, three products are sold over the counter in the UK – comfort milk, anti-reflux milk and lactose-free formula – and these products add to the confusion families feel about the type of milk they should use. These should not be sold over the counter as there are a number of issues which make them less suitable for most infants than infant formula. This category also includes milks which are available on prescription for specific medical conditions.

Toddler milks and 'growing up milks' are used by companies to extend their product reach by making it appear that your child moves from stage 1 to stage 2, 3 and 4 formula. If children are not breastfed after 1 year of age (and breastmilk remains the best choice of main milk drink throughout the second year of life) then they can move to whole animal milk or a suitable alternative as their main milk drink. Toddler milks are not regulated in any way but use the same branding which cross-promotes other products in advertising.

Supporting families with normal, healthy infants and young children

Questions you may be asked about breastmilk substitutes and sources of information about products on the UK market

Will hungry baby formula help a baby sleep better?

No. There is no evidence that milks marketed for hungry babies offer any advantage, and it is recommended that first whey-based infant formula are used throughout the first year of life if babies are not being breastfed.

Is formula based on goats' milk less allergenic than formula made from cows' milk?

No. Milk-based infant formula can have cows' milk or goats' milk protein as the main protein source. They are equivalent in terms of allergenicity and safety.

Is soya-based formula a good option if there are allergies in the family or if families are vegetarian?

No. Soya-based formula is not recommended for use in infants under 6 months of age unless recommended by a medical practitioner. These milks are not recommended for use without medical supervision for a number of reasons (see box).

> Children are as likely to be allergic to soya as to cows' milk protein, and this needs to be investigated. Soya is a rich source of phyto-oestrogens and these mimic sex hormones in the body. For older children and adults, some soya is not a problem, but for babies under 6 months who have soya protein-based formula as their sole source of nutrition, current guidance in the UK is that the phyto-oestrogens in soya-based formula should be carefully considered as a risk. The carbohydrate source of soya protein-based formula is maltodextrin, which is more likely to damage teeth.
>
> If infants are allergic to cows' milk, they will be prescribed a suitable formula by their GP, and it is recommended that parents and carers should not use soya formula without taking professional medical advice.

Are ready-to-feed milks different to powdered milks?

There are some small compositional differences between powdered and ready-to-feed milks, but there is little information available as to whether these are of any significance. Current evidence does not support anecdotal ideas that ready-to-feed milks are 'easier to digest'. Ready-to-feed milks are less likely to be halal-approved than powdered formulations. Ready-to-feed milks are also much more expensive than powdered milks, particularly when sold in 'starter kit' 70-mL bottles. Ready-to-feed milks also require considerably more packaging, which has an impact on the environment.

What non-dairy alternatives to cows' milk are suitable from 1 year of age?

Any whole animal milk is suitable as the main drink from 1 year of age – cows', goats' or sheep's milk, as long as these are pasteurised. An unsweetened calcium-fortified soya milk alternative, oat milk alternative, hemp milk alternative or pea- or nut-based

Table 17.1 A simple guide to choosing milks as the main milk drink for most infants and toddlers

Type of milk	Infants 0–6 months	Infants 6 months–1 year	Toddlers 1–2 years
Breastmilk	✓	✓	✓
Whole cows' milk (or goats' milk, sheep's milk)	✗	✗	✓
Infant formula suitable from birth (cows' or goats' milk-based)	✓	✓	Not needed
Soya protein-based infant formula suitable from birth	Only use under medical supervision	Only use under medical supervision	Not needed
Infant formula marketed for hungrier babies, suitable from birth (cows' milk-based)	Not recommended	Not recommended	Not needed
Follow-on formula suitable from 6 months of age (cows' or goats' milk-based)	✗	Not recommended	Not needed
Goodnight milk	✗	Not recommended	Not needed
Growing-up milks and toddler milks suitable from around 1 year of age (cows' milk, goats' milk or soya milk-based)	✗	✗	Not needed
Unsweetened calcium-fortified soya milk alternative or other unsweetened fortified milk alternatives as main milk drink. N.B.: Milk alternatives are low in energy and can be low in protein and should be used carefully in the diets of very young children	✗	✗	✓
Rice milk alternative – do not give to children under 5 years of age	✗	✗	✗

✓ = Safe to give; ✗ = do not give this milk.

milk alternative can be given (these can also be called soya drink, oat drink, and so on). However, care needs to be taken if milk alternatives are used for children under 5 that the diet is energy- and nutrient-dense as milk alternatives are lower in energy and most are lower in protein. Some milk alternatives do not provide important nutrients such as riboflavin and iodine that animal milks provide. Rice milk alternative (also called rice milk drink) should not be given to infants or children under 5. For information on non-dairy sources of calcium and milk alternatives to choose for children who avoid dairy products, see *Eating well: vegan infants and under-5s*, available from www.firststepsnutrition.org

Is an infant milk for 'fussy eaters' useful?

Periods of fussy eating are common in young children and in most cases resolve themselves if families continue to offer a range of foods, eat with their children and act as a good role model for eating a range of foods. Occasionally a child will have a more serious case of food refusal, and advice should be sought on how to manage this most effectively. Giving a fussy child a sweet milkshake drink (such as Pediasure shake) will not help them eat better in the long term, and we discourage the use of any fortified milks for this purpose unless they are used under medical supervision.

Supporting families where an infant may need a specialist formula

If a baby is bringing up milk after feeds, does s/he need a special formula to prevent reflux?

Many babies will bring up small amounts of milk after feeds or if they burp, and this causes them no distress. Crying, vomiting milk after feeds and arching the back or being unsettled are not symptoms of reflux in most babies. Reflux is rare and should be properly diagnosed by a paediatrician. If a baby brings up milk after feeds, it may be that s/he needs smaller milk feeds more often or may need more frequent winding during a feed. Using responsive bottlefeeding techniques will lead to far fewer incidences of perceived reflux. Thickened (anti-reflux) milks should only be used under medical supervision but can be purchased over the counter in the UK. There are several reasons to be cautious about using these milks:

- These formulas contain cereal-based thickeners, and are higher in protein than infant formula. Higher-protein intakes are now being linked to later adiposity.
- Manufacturers recommend that anti-reflux formula are made up at lower temperatures than the temperature currently recommended for safety, and it is important that this potential risk is considered by a medical practitioner. Powdered infant formulas are not sterile and making them up at lower temperatures will not kill any harmful bacteria that might be present.
- If a baby is taking certain medicines, it may not be advisable to give him or her an anti-reflux formula.

National Institute of Health and Clinical Excellence (NICE) guidelines are available to support health professionals: www.nice.org.uk/guidance/ng1/resources/gastrooesophageal-reflux-disease-recognition-diagnosis-and-management-in-children-and-young-people-51035086789. This guidance has also been reiterated in NICE Quality Standards, published in 2016, available at www.nice.org.uk/guidance/qs112

Powdered infant milks are not sterile and they may contain harmful bacteria such as *Salmonella* and *Cronobacter sakazakii*, but a range of *Cronobacter* species can be present in powdered infant milks. The key recommendation from all international bodies to reduce risk to infants from bacterial infection has been to encourage the reconstitution of infant formula with water at no less than 70°C. Clear advice on making up infant milks safely can be found at www.unicef.org.uk/babyfriendly/wp-content/uploads/sites/2/2008/02/start4life_guide_to_bottle_-feeding.pdf

Will a comfort milk reduce colic?

No. It is not uncommon for young babies to be unsettled or fussy in the evenings and to cry more than they might at other times of the day. The average amount a baby cries in the first 6 weeks of life is about 110 minutes a day, reducing to about 75 minutes a day at 10–12 weeks. All babies are different and many need more attention and soothing in the evenings, frequent small feeds and frequent winding (during and after feeds) in the first few months. There is no consistent evidence that comfort milks improve babies' wind, colic, constipation or fussiness, and these will pass as the baby gets older. Often small changes to the timing and quantity of feeds can be effective in managing periods of fussiness.

If a baby has diarrhoea and looks in pain after feeds, is a lactose-free formula useful?

Lactose intolerance is rare in babies, and symptoms associated with lactose intolerance may also suggest cows' milk protein allergy. Cows' milk protein allergy is also uncommon but, if a baby has sickness or diarrhoea, signs of an immediate allergic reaction after a milk feed (a red itchy rash around the mouth, facial swelling, red lumps on the body or a streaming nose) or symptoms of a delayed reaction such as eczema or poor growth, it is important to get a proper diagnosis. Diarrhoea may be a symptom of a gastrointestinal infection rather than an intolerance, and some babies might have a temporary lactose intolerance after a bout of gastrointestinal illness. It is important lactose-free milks are only used under medical supervision, as the source of carbohydrate in these milks is more likely to damage teeth and the risks of using any specialist milk products should always be weighed up against any potential benefit.

How do we manage suspected allergy to cows' milk protein?

Breastfeeding is the best way to protect a baby from developing allergies and cows' milk protein allergy is rare in breastfed babies. If there is suspected cows' milk protein allergy in a breastfed infant then maternal exclusion of cows' milk protein is the first line of action. Cows' milk protein allergy is uncommon (less than 2% of UK infants). Revised guidance on the diagnosis and management of cows' milk protein allergy (called the iMAP guidance) has taken into consideration previous criticisms that it led to overdiagnosis and provides better support to maintain the breastfeeding relationship. This is available from the GP Infant Feeding Network (GPIFN: www.gpifn. org.uk).

The majority of infants diagnosed with cows' milk protein allergy will require an extensively hydrolysed formula (which is prescribable and costs about £20/800 g). Very few will need an amino acid-based formula but these are heavily marketed as first-line treatment (although they often cost £60/800 g). For details of all specialist milks on the UK market suitable for infants see *Specialised Infant Milks in the UK* at www.firststepsnutrition.org/composition-claims-and-cost.

One brand of infant formula claims to reduce the risk of a baby developing an allergy, but experts in the UK do not believe there is good enough evidence to make this claim.

References

WHO (1981) *International Code of Marketing of Breast-Milk Substitutes*. Geneva: WHO. www.who.int/nutrition/publications/code_english.pdf

WHO (2017) *The International Code of Marketing of Breast-Milk Substitutes – 2017 Update. Frequently Asked Questions*. Geneva: WHO. https://apps.who.int/iris/bitstream/handle/10665/254911/WHO-NMH-NHD-17.1-eng.pdf?ua=1

18 Stopping breastfeeding

Emma Pickett

For some mothers, breastfeeding has been difficult, and the ending of breastfeeding is something they eagerly anticipate. For other families, breastfeeding has been at the core of a positive parenting experience. It has been far more than a milk delivery system, but a valued tool used throughout their parenting. In line with World Health Organization recommendations, breastfeeding may have continued for 2 years and beyond. The ending of breastfeeding can be an emotional time for both the child and parent. Breastfeeding may sometimes end at the child's discretion. If child-led weaning does occur, it will often happen between 2 and 5 years. However, in our culture, breastfeeding will often be mother-led. Whichever way breastfeeding ends, it's important to acknowledge that powerful hormones are involved and some mothers experience grief and loss when they were least expecting to. Breastfeeding should end gradually to allow supply to diminish safely and to reduce risks of blocked ducts, mastitis and abscesses. This will also allow both mother and child to make an emotional adjustment and establish an alternative feeding method.

Unsurprisingly, the decision on whether to stop breastfeeding is ideally something that happens happily. If the mother appears to choose to end breastfeeding, this may still not be a decision she is entirely comfortable with. Family and cultural pressure, especially when feeding an older child, can lead mums to end breastfeeding reluctantly. When we know that breastfeeding has a protective effect on maternal mental health, this could have serious implications (Brown 2018). Breastfeeding peer supporters may be able to support the mother to have conversations with family and close friends if she does wish to continue.

If a mother has been told that she needs to end breastfeeding in order to have medical treatment or to take medications, this is something that will need careful research. If a drug is deemed to be unsafe, an alternative can often be found. For mothers with a history of mental health issues, it is particularly important that they are supported to breastfeed for as long as they wish. Research suggests that ending breastfeeding does not improve maternal sleep (Montgomery-Downs et al. 2010). For mothers who are struggling, breastfeeding can be the one thing they feel they can do successfully.

Some mothers may be nervous about breastfeeding on a return to work. A conversation with a peer supporter, breastfeeding counsellor or lactation consultant can give her practical tips which can help to make continued breastfeeding possible and it may even make the transition to returning to work easier for baby and mother.

When we are confident that the mother does wish to end breastfeeding, there are some basic principles that will apply in all cases. Even if a mother does need to end breastfeeding in an urgent situation, she would still ideally continue expressing for at least a few more days to gradually reduce the demand from the breast and send messages to begin the shutdown of production. When mothers do end breastfeeding, we are looking to avoid engorgement which can lead to discomfort and, in some cases, mastitis. When mothers are ending breastfeeding after a longer period, they may have fewer physical symptoms and experience no engorgement at all. If mothers have been feeding a younger baby more frequently, even if they follow the recommendation to take 2 or 3 days between dropping each feed, they may still experience some fullness. This may sometimes be described as lumpiness but these lumps can be glandular tissue at full storage capacity rather than a blocked duct or something that requires treatment. If the tenderness is localised and mastitis symptoms develop, then it may be the process of ending breastfeeding is delayed as mastitis treatment takes place.

It is normal for a mother to continue to see evidence of milk for several weeks after the last feed. This can sometimes be upsetting for mothers, but they can be reassured that involution of breast tissue can commonly take more than a month. The urge to check if milk is still present will continue stimulation. It is not recommended to bind or compress the breast as part of the weaning process.

If a baby is under 12 months, the family will need information on safe formula preparation. Follow-on milk is not required and first formula is suitable for the first 12 months. Responsive bottlefeeding is recommended to reduce risk of overfeeding and feeding can continue as an opportunity for cuddles and bonding with primary caregivers.

If parents are struggling to encourage a baby to take a bottle for the first time, a health visitor or a local feeding drop-in may be able to give support. Sometimes offering a bottle after a short breastfeed when the baby is more relaxed will encourage greater acceptance. Some babies will only accept a bottle when they are hungrier. There is a lot of individual variation. Many families will be told that one particular bottle is more likely to be accepted or is 'closer to breastfeeding' and this is a group of parents who are particularly vulnerable to manipulation by advertising and promotion.

A baby who is between 6 and 12 months old, especially one who has taken to solid food enthusiastically, may be able to avoid the use of bottles entirely and move to having formula milk in a cup. After 12 months, full-fat cows' milk can be given and formula is no longer necessary. Occasionally, an older child who has been breastfeeding happily may be reluctant to drink milk in another form. If water is given in a cup alongside a diet rich in dairy or equivalent products, this does not necessarily pose a problem.

Of course, breastfeeding is only partially about milk. For both the child and mother there is an emotional and relationship-building element that needs to be considered as part of the weaning process. A conscious effort to make feeding still a time for closeness, cuddling and eye contact is important. Babies may feel more unsettled as often breastfeeding has comforted them when they are feeling tired or overstimulated.

Mothers can also be surprised at the sense of loss that can come with the end of breastfeeding, even when it is something they had full control over. The hormonal shifts will affect some women more than others. It can also bring up emotions about the entire breastfeeding journey and it's important that mothers are supported and have an opportunity to speak to someone who understands and has time to listen.

For many, it is far from simply a practical process of swapping from one method of feeding to another.

With older children, the method, 'Don't offer, don't refuse', is often suggested. However, for some toddlers and pre-schoolers this will not bring a rapid end to breastfeeding. If breastfeeding is intertwined with sleep, the family may require more support. After years of gentle parenting, leaving a toddler and pre-schooler to cry is often something that breastfeeding families feel uncomfortable doing. Sleep habits can be improved in a variety of ways which can bring an easier end to a long positive breastfeeding experience. Removing the mother from the situation and substituting other family members may not be sensible when for the child the loss is not simply one of breastfeeding, but of the close connection with the breast owner. It can take time for an older child to learn to fall asleep and to transition between sleep cycles overnight without the breast. While breastfeeding does not increase the risk of dental caries, introducing a bottle at bedtime and overnight can. Parents may need support to develop new techniques which prepare a child to fall asleep comfortably. This may be close contact, singing a gentle song, the use of recorded music or white noise. Some children enthusiastically accept a transitional object such as a cuddly toy.

During the day, a request for a breastfeed is ideally avoided so that refusal is not needed. For many older children the importance of their request being met and the opportunity for undivided attention are powerful. It may be that choosing and reading a book together is a more suitable substitute for a breastfeed than a cup of milk. Older children can often be distracted when a breastfeeding request appears imminent and when breastfeeding is associated with a particular time of day or a particular chair, changing schedules even for just a few days can reduce the amount of breastfeeding that happens.

Even when breastfeeding has only occurred for a few days, weeks or months, mothers should be supported to end breastfeeding whenever they wish to do so. Mothers are often hard on themselves and encouraging them to find support and treat themselves with kindness during this difficult time is very important. Breastfeeding should ideally always end gradually to allow for an emotional adjustment and also to give breasts time to reduce milk supply and reduce the risk of breast problems.

References

Brown A (2018) What do women lose if they are prevented from meeting their breastfeeding goals? *Clin Lactat* 9(4):200–7.

Montgomery-Downs HE, Clawges HM, Santy EE (2010) Infant feeding methods and maternal sleep and daytime functioning. *Pediatrics* 126:e1562.

19 Where to find out more

For further information and support you can contact any of the breastfeeding organisations as a professional

Nation Breastfeeding Helpline – 0300 100 0212
Association of Breastfeeding Mothers – 0300 330 5453
La Leche League – 0345 120 2918
National Childbirth Trust (NCT) – 0300 330 0700

For information on medications and breastmilk

Breastfeeding Network Drugs in Breastmilk Service: www.breastfeedingnetwork.org.uk/detailed-information/drugs-in-breastmilk
UK Drugs in Lactation Advisory Service (UKDILAS): www.sps.nhs.uk/articles/ukdilas
Breastfeeding and Medication: http://breastfeeding-and-medication.co.uk

For further impartial advice around formula supplementation

First Steps Nutrition Trust: www.firststepsnutrition.org

For further education and training

Unicef UK Baby Friendly Initiative training for paediatricians and GPs: www.unicef.org.uk/babyfriendly/training/e-learning
GP Infant Feeding Network: https://gpifn.org.uk

For further information and reading around breastfeeding

Unicef UK Baby Friendly Initiative: www.unicef.org.uk/babyfriendly
Breastfeeding Network: www.breastfeedingnetwork.org.uk
Association of Breastfeeding Mothers: https://abm.me.uk
La Leche League: www.laleche.org.uk
National Childbirth Trust (NCT): www.nct.org.uk
Human Milk Foundation: https://humanmilkfoundation.org

Centre for Lactation, Infant Feeding and Translation: www.swansea.ac.uk/
humanandhealthsciences/research-at-the-college-of-human-and-health/
research-centres-and-groups-at-human-and-health/lactation-infant-feeding-
translational-research/
Baby Sleep Information Source: www.basisonline.org.uk

Further recommended reading

Brown A (2016) *Breastfeeding Uncovered*. Pinter and Martin.
Brown A (2017) *Why Starting Solids Matters*. Pinter and Martin.
Brown A (2018) *The Positive Breastfeeding Book*. Pinter and Martin.
Jones W (2016) *The Importance of Dads and Grandmas to the Breastfeeding Mothers*.
Praeclarus Press.
Jones W (2017) *Why Mother's Medication Matters*. Pinter and Martin.
Jones W (2018) *Breastfeeding and Medication* (2nd ed). Routledge.
Kendall-Tackett K (ed.) (2018) *Promoting Breastfeeding: Medical Settings*. Praeclarus Press.
Lawrence RA, Lawrence RM (2011) *Breastfeeding: A Guide for the Medical Profession*.
Elsevier Health Sciences.
Newman J, Pitman T (2014) *Dr Jack Newman's Guide to Breastfeeding*. Pinter and Martin.

Index

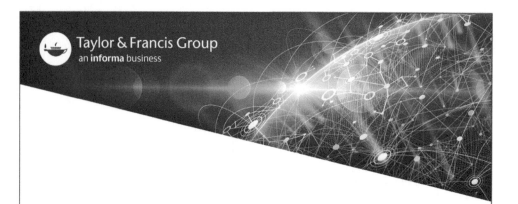
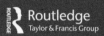
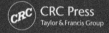